Healing the Power in You

Tapping into Courage, Hope, and Resilience

Joalie Davie, MD

Health from Within Books
Santa Fe, NM

Praise

"This is a magnificent book. Joalie Davie, a Harvard- and U-Mass. Medical School-trained physician, has passed through the eye of the needle to attain true healing wisdom. Drawing on her personal medical challenges, she learned to combine the best that medical science has to offer with consciousness-oriented techniques that are too often neglected by conventional physicians. The result is an advanced form of healing that, quite simply, *works*. As you read these fascinating case histories, be aware that you are witnessing the medicine of the future. Buy two copies: one for you and one for your doctor."

~ Larry Dossey, MD, *New York Times* best-selling author of *One Mind: How Our Individual Mind Is Part of a Greater Consciousness and Why It Matters* and other books; executive editor of *Explore: The Journal of Science and Healing*

"Dr. Davie's book is full of wisdom. And what is wisdom? It is knowledge tempered by experience. It is intellect tempered with heart. Dr. Davie's very clear commitment is to discover what works and offer that to her patients. She is willing to travel into arenas not normally explored by traditional medicine to discover additional doorways into healing."

~ Martin Rutte, founder of Project Heaven on Earth; co-author of the *New York Times* best-seller *Chicken Soup for the Soul at Work*

"*Healing the Power in You* is a must-read for anyone interested in achieving optimum health—a blueprint for using the brain to turn physical and psychological obstacles into stepping stones. It is a new paradigm for healing. The message is powerful: we have the answers within us. She documents cures that she's facilitated through alternative modalities, such as the removal of a neck tumor, overcoming ACE (Adverse Childhood Experience), even overcoming cancer. Each chapter ends with exercises for tapping into one's own power to heal. The appendices offer valuable suggestions, from an anti-inflammatory diet to notes on Eye Movement Desensitization and Reprocessing (EMDR), hypnosis, and a multitude of approaches to wellness. The tone of *Healing the Power in You* is friendly, compassionate, and lively. This book is a gem, not to be missed."

~ Elaine Pinkerton, author of seven books, including
Santa Fe on Foot

"Compelling, personal, and informative, Dr. Joalie Davie's book shows how conventional medical practice addresses only the body, instead of a whole body-mind-spirit combination. Her emphasis on the importance of childhood trauma is so essential, but many physicians miss this factor. By using energy psychology techniques to quickly resolve the emotional underpinnings of medical issues, as well as spiritual practices of love and forgiveness, she empowers the inner healer in each patient to flourish."

~ Barbara Stone, PhD, author of *Invisible Roots*
and *Transforming Fear into Gold*; originator of
SoulDetective.net

"Dr. Joalie is compassionate, insightful, and intuitive. She listens closely to patients and possesses the skills to ask the right question at the right time. The result is a true shift in perspective: negative feelings that had seemed so impossible to shake, are lifted; feelings of hopelessness are replaced with a sense of optimism and peace. No one could ask for a more skilled and caring therapist."

~ Christine Farrell-Riley, MD

Published by: Health from Within Books
PO Box 23293
Santa Fe, NM 87504
www.healthfromwithin.com

ISBN 978-1-947982-00-0 (paperback); 978-1-947982-01-7 (audio/mp3); 978-1-947982-02-4 (mobi); 978-1-947982-03-1 (epub)

Library of Congress Control Number: 2018909554

Publisher's Cataloging-in-Publication Data
Names: Davie, Joalie
Title: Healing the power in you: tapping into courage, hope, and resilience
Description: Santa Fe: Health from Within Books, 2018. | Includes bibliographical references, glossary, and diagrams
Identifiers: LCCN 2018909554 | ISBN 9781947982000 (paper) | ISBN 9781947982017 (audio) | ISBN 9781947982024 (mobi) | ISBN 9781947982031 (epub)
Subjects: 1. Healing--psychological aspects. 2. Holistic medicine. 3. Self-care, Health. 4. Mind and body--therapies. 5. Stress management. 6. Medicine--case studies. I. Davie, Joalie II. Title.
Classification: R733 .D 2018 | DDC 615.5—dc23

Cover photograph © 2018 Joalie Davie

Cover design by Leslie Waltzer, Crowfoot Designs

Printed in the United States of America

10 09 08 07 06 05 04 03 02 01

Disclaimer

My work with people differs from standard medical interventions and does not replace the need for conventional medical care. No one should embark on complementary techniques without informing his or her doctor. This book is not intended as a substitute for medical advice from physicians.

The work I do supports and complements other doctors' treatment plans. I provide information on medical and other research to educate individuals about some of the various options available and to help them make an informed decision when discussing issues with their primary care providers.

I encourage readers to take responsibility for their well-being and healing and to enlist the help and support of a competent healthcare team, which may include a primary care provider and medical specialists, as well as a psychologist and/or health coach. An abundance of effective healing techniques exists; no single person can be aware of them all. A partial list of resources mentioned in this book is included in Appendix D. Professionals on your team should be attuned to mind/body/spirit wellness and fully versed in the techniques you explore.

The information provided in this book is intended for your general knowledge only and is not a substitute for professional medical advice or treatment for specific medical conditions. The reader should not use this information to diagnose or treat a health problem or disease without consulting a qualified healthcare provider.

Never disregard professional medical advice or delay in seeking it because of something stated in this book. This book does not teach or recommend any specific approach, nor is it meant to replace sound medical advice or treatment programs.

References to clinical studies and diagrams of postures commonly used in this work are also appended.

I wrote this book for you, the reader

    who looks for answers,

    who asks questions,

    who questions answers,

    who is willing to explore possibilities and solutions

    for health and wellness.

To my mother for her love, dedication, and support

To my teachers, my patients, my students, and readers

Contents

Acknowledgments

There are several individuals whose inspiration and contributions made this book possible.

I thank my editor, Mary Neighbour, for challenging me to write about my personal experience and articulate my feelings and opinions. I appreciate her patience and ability to see through the words the deeper meanings that need to be expressed.

I am grateful to my patients for their stories, their trust, their courage, and their commitment to health. They are teachers to everyone who reads this book, as they were my teachers in the work we did. I especially thank those individuals who asked that I use their real names in my book: Rhea, Carlos, and Christopher. (All other names and some personal details have been changed to protect individual privacy and identity.)

I am grateful to my students who have also been my teachers, showing me even more ways to heal.

I am grateful to my teachers in medical school, specifically Israel Abroms, fondly known as Kuna, for knowing and demonstrating that the human body's healing capacity is limitless and beyond medical understanding, that children expand the medical understanding of the human potential.

I am grateful to the many friends and others who guided my journey of discovery, learning, and transformation at the Milton Erickson Foundation, the Focusing Institute, the National Institute for the Clinical Application of Behavioral Medicine (NICABM), the Association for Comprehensive Energy Psychology (ACEP), and the Canadian Association for Integrative and Energy Therapies (CAIET).

I am grateful to Sandi Radomski and her colleagues, Tom and Pam Altaffer, for their support and generosity in allowing me to share the statements of Ask and Receive.

I am grateful to my family for their support and consideration: my mother for reading and commenting on the manuscript; my sister, Eliane, and brother-in-law, Gary, for their advice and assistance; and my brother, Jacques, for his heartfelt encouragement.

I am grateful to my daughter, Michelle, for diagrams in Appendix B and for her input and helpful insights.

I am grateful for the generosity and support of Gregg Braden (bestselling, award-winning author) for sharing his wisdom.

I am grateful to Martin Rutte, co-author of *Chicken Soup for the Soul* and creator of Heaven on Earth, for his support and generosity.

I am grateful to my friends and colleagues, Bruce Patterson and Christine Farrell-Riley, for their support and encouragement.

I am grateful for living in a beautiful state with glorious sunrises, sunsets, skies, and mountains.

I am grateful to you, the reader. My wish is that you will be inspired to explore new possibilities for healing that will improve your well-being, happiness, and life. Courage, hope, and resilience make health and wellness possible.

Foreword

Some stories need to be told because it is important for the teller to tell them; others need to be told because the world needs to hear them. This book is full of the latter. I do not consider it an exaggeration to say that its contents can reasonably restore hope in those who have been disappointed, sometimes devastatingly, by the limitations of Western-only medicine.

There remains in Western medical culture a widespread assumption that seems to me as tragic as it is astounding, nearly two decades into the twenty-first century: i.e., that whatever is happening in a person's body has nothing to do with what is happening in that person's life. This assumption leads almost all healing enquiry into the *why* of a condition while ignoring the whole-person (holistic) question of *why now?*

With the keen mind and voracious curiosity of a born scientist, Dr. Davie's investigations of complementary- and alternative-healing practices have led to exciting, life-changing and life-saving discoveries, precisely because they address the question of *why now?* She explores this question from angles too many physicians do not, or do not want to, see. And trusting her own experience, even when it flew in the face of what she'd been taught or told, is how this remarkable doctor arrived at the surprising successes revealed here.

I met Dr. Davie years ago at a Focusing training; we both were practitioners and students of energy psychology. I didn't know at the time that she was also a rigorously trained, Harvard-educated physician who had learned the hard way that to restore health— her patients' or her own—she had no choice but to think outside the box. If necessity is the mother of invention, it may also be the mother of discovery and synthesis, as Dr. Joalie's personal odyssey back to health, and that of each patient described in these pages, demonstrates.

As a trauma therapist, I can attest to the unique characteristics of medical traumas. Trips to the dentist may turn into traumas of bodily invasion and parental betrayal, the symptoms of which can mimic those of childhood sexual abuse. Similarly, mechanically and impersonally imposed medical treatments and procedures can re-traumatize a person, while only treating the symptom, not the cause, of the problem.

Having learned through experience to avoid such mistakes, Dr. Davie is able to help her patients connect to and activate their inherent capacity to self-heal, and to access that knowing place within, something all healthcare providers would do well to elicit and listen to.

I speak from personal experience, for my friend has treated me with the same success that you will find in these stories. She uncovers, addresses, and resolves the roots of problems that baffle us on the surface—and faster than we used to think possible.

Dr. Joalie's tenacious, hard-to-prove conviction that there must be something *more*, something *else* that can help, is in itself a belief with the power to heal. It leads to our capacity to self-heal (often with some outside assistance). If ever there was an empowering belief worthy of contagion, surely this qualifies. Perhaps you'll catch it by reading this inspiring book and find in its pages, as I have, the voice of hope itself.

Bruce Patterson, LCSW
New York City

Postscript: Don't just *read* the exercises at the end of each chapter—*do* them. If you're like me and learn best by trying something yourself, you'll experience what she's talking about on a deeper level.

Introduction

Finding Wellness through Pain and Trauma

Remember: The entrance door to the
sanctuary is inside you. – Rumi

ONLY MY EYES and my vocal cords could move. Trapped and held tight by a giant male orderly, I screamed with all my nine-year-old might as tears ran down my face. I had trusted the otolaryngologist, the husband of a dear aunt, when he promised he would only remove two bits of tissue from my throat. But he did not stop. He reached again into my mouth, stretched wide by a metal instrument, and plucked a third piece of bloody pulp. I did not recognize my sweet, obedient self as I let out another outraged shriek.

The tonsillectomy must have lasted less than ten minutes, but to me it seemed like an hour. Even though I experienced no physical pain, I felt I had been assaulted and cut up in a most cruel way. Afterward, sitting on the couch in a cozy room, my mom and my aunt chatted cheerfully and tried to console me, entreating me with ice cream. Angry and crying, I felt no pleasure in eating this rare treat.

As many readers will recognize, that is the effect of shocking ordeals: they eclipse joy and reality and isolate you in a shadowy realm of fear and vulnerability. Although pain during medical treatments cannot always be avoided, attention should be given to minimizing traumatic consequences. As a physician, I know my profession can do better. It requires more compassion and understanding. We must listen and believe what the patient presents as their own truth.

In the following case studies from my practice, I describe people who have experienced the shortcomings of modern medicine—including the fallibility of procedures, pharmaceuticals, and the practitioners of Western medicine. Individuals come to me seeking alternatives that can restore them to health. Many are astonished by the journey to reclaimed well-being; it is not far in the distance or elusive. Health and wholeness reside within each of us.

In the following stories you will witness real-life transformations. I include my own tortuous experiences, which stretched throughout my young adulthood and training at Harvard and the University of Massachusetts Medical School. Yes, I was one of those practitioners, steeped in Western traditions of healing. I expected my body to respond like a machine, and when it didn't, my doctors and I blamed my body: it was resistant! I wore blinders for many years to the insidious effects of emotional traumas I had experienced, and I sometimes took for granted the remarkable, innate human capacity for recuperation, repair, and restoration.

My transition from a narrow perspective on health and healing to a broad and refreshing view of wellness is explained in Chapter 1, "Joalie: A Journey from Cynicism to Skepticism to Practitioner of Alternative and Integrative Medicine." Each of the following chapters explores well-being in the context of various common ailments, such as heart disease, obesity, PTSD, and depression. I introduce a variety of alternative, integrative, complementary modalities, describe outcomes, and discuss the possible dynamics at work. After each chapter, I offer a simple exercise that I hope will inspire you to consider exploring different techniques as steppingstones to your own healing. A glossary at the back of this book will help define some of the practices I use and related terminology.

Lives have been saved—and what appears at first to be a medical miracle will become comprehensible and attainable by the time you finish reading. The possibilities for physical and emotional well-being are limitless, and they are accessible. Alternative, integrative, and complementary practices will soon be the standard of care.

My goal in writing this book is to bring to your awareness some of these choices, which offer a new paradigm for health and healing. My intention is to extend hope to those who feel hopeless, courage to those who are afraid, and belief and understanding to those who have lost faith in being well. With each case study you will see how ordinary people find within themselves the power to heal. You, too, can find and manifest this power.

Chapter 1: Joalie

A Journey from Cynicism to Skepticism to Practitioner of Alternative and Integrative Medicine

Until you are willing to be confused about what you already know, what you know will never grow bigger, better, or more useful. – Milton Erickson, MD

IN CONVENTIONAL MEDICINE, physicians typically develop a diagnosis and then work to confirm or disprove it, relying heavily on lab tests, physical findings, drugs, and surgeries. While the patient's history and presentation are also considered, the diagnosis is limited to what is known and determined by the established fund of knowledge. When patients do not respond as expected, then they may be considered a dilemma and sometimes a hypochondriac. However, a diagnosis is not—and must not be—as important as the outcome of restored health, and considerations of many aspects of a person's life should be taken into account.

I did not always think this way. After my tonsillectomy at age nine, I appreciated that the surgery successfully stopped my recurrent bouts of bronchitis and sinusitis. I valued my health, ate consciously, and believed my vigorous exercise, with a good, clean sweat, helped defeat colds and other infections. I remained healthy and physically active through my teens and twenties and no longer missed weeks of school in the winter.

Following in my grandfather's footsteps, I became a doctor. Educated at Harvard and the University of Massachusetts Medical School, I worked for twelve years in emergency and internal medicine and became known as an erudite and skilled professional. If anyone thirty years ago had said that today I would be practicing alternative and integrative medicine—which I am—I would have thought it the most preposterous idea. Beyond being cynical, I believed anything but conventional Western medicine was pure quackery.

What caused my transformation and brought me to the exploration of alternative healing? It all began in early adulthood with the reemergence of bronchitis and sinusitis: three to four times a year, increasing to six to eight annually. As these infections became more frequent, they became more tenacious and resistant to usual treatments. I progressed from using standard to broad-spectrum antibiotics and then to needing second- and third-generation antibiotics. By 1990, even these were no longer effective. Cipro, a newer drug, worked for about a year, until I developed a severe infection that would not clear with any drug on the market. I couldn't breathe through my nose, and the disorder interfered with my healthy, active life.

The story that follows—about my pursuit of health—is just one of millions of medical ordeals, which real people all over the world have endured. The plot twists include inaccessibility of care, incompetence of apathetic practitioners, my own, very human

2

need to believe in a cure, and my absolute faith in the infallibility of conventional medicine.

Though I sometimes felt alone, I was not. I benefited from competent, caring doctors who, like me, regarded standard medicine as the only option. I received professional and compassionate attention from my internist and infectious disease consultant, for which I am deeply grateful.

Along this path, many assurances were made and later dashed. In the care of a series of esteemed and recommended specialists, I underwent numerous consultations, assessments, and treatments. I received multiple diagnoses but no relief. To the contrary, my condition deteriorated, and I also developed additional maladies, many worse than the original condition for which I was being treated.

The memory of my tonsillectomy left me with an aversion to further surgery. However, I had run out of options and consented to a sinus operation. I tried to reason away my anxiety and focus on the prospect the treatment would again take care of all my problems. Indeed, when discharged I received a glowing prognosis, even though my nasal passages and face were so swollen I couldn't breathe through my nose or smell anything.

For two days I felt hopeful. I ignored my intuition that something was seriously wrong. My otolaryngologist was the expert. How could I doubt his opinion? Like many, I accepted his authority without questioning. When a bloody, foul-smelling discharge developed, however, dismay and anxiety prompted me to call the surgeon, now on vacation. The covering doctor examined me and discovered a loose piece of bone stuck in my nasal cavity. I expected its removal would clear the problem, but within a week, I ran a high fever with a thick discharge. Now both surgeons were unavailable, so I saw my internist. She cultured the drainage and put me on antibiotics once more.

Eventually I obtained a follow-up with the original surgeon. Even though I felt awful, he proclaimed everything looked fine. To my horror, after examining me with a scope, he merely wiped it with alcohol and placed it in its case. I asked him if he had properly sterilized it before using it on me, and he admitted he hadn't. I asked him what the recommendations were, and he said the scope needed to be soaked for ten minutes in a solution and then autoclaved, but he only did so once a week—to protect the instrument. I felt a hole in my gut! He cared about his instruments and wallet more than his patients. Extremely upset, I just wanted out of his office, never to return. However, I remained cordial, as I always was to other physicians, and I even thanked him.

Burying my feelings, I met with yet another specialist. I staggered through six ENT (Ear-Nose-Throat) consultations. All but one of these recommended surgery to remove the swollen tissue. I could not understand what was happening to me. Nothing made sense. The offending inflammation and tissue were removed—why didn't I heal like a case study in the medical books? I wanted an explanation. I needed a doctor to believe in and a treatment that would take care of my sinus problem, and my fatigue, so I could return to working sixty hours a week. I wanted to run and cycle and do aerobics and continue my life.

Desperate for a solution, believing a "fix" lay just around the corner, I did not give up. Wearily, I continued my search and eventually agreed to a second surgery. To prepare myself and be as healthy as possible before the procedure, I went to the ocean. I walked on the beach, bicycled, swam, read, and I ate wholesome, home-cooked meals. By the time I returned home, I felt much better. My sinuses were clear, and I was 70 percent back to my old self.

Did I still need the surgery? The compliant, obedient part of me decided to trust my doctor would do the right thing, as he promised. On the day of the operation, I let him know how I prepared for it and now felt much better, though not yet 100 percent. Smiling, he said in a paternalistic tone that he would take care of everything.

The next thing I remember is waking up, groggy, with a horrific headache and severe swelling, as if my face were going to explode. I knew at the very core of my being that something was terribly wrong. Drained, as if life itself had been extracted from me, I fought against scary thoughts: was that cerebrospinal fluid oozing from my nasal passages? I tasted the liquid to make sure it was not sweet; it seemed salty, but I remained concerned. Was my brain compromised?

Regretting I had subjected myself to the surgeries, I nevertheless held fast to the illusion that *good* medicine would and could resolve my health issues. I returned to the surgeon, but he ignored my symptoms and told me nothing was wrong. "Eat more," he advised. I felt betrayed and abandoned by a medical profession that would not take responsibility for its failures.

Fortunately I could rely on my internist, who was dependable, compassionate, and doing her best. She cultured my infection, tested for effective antibiotics, and prescribed them. The results showed that now multi-drug-resistant *Pseudomonas, Aeruginosa,* and *Klebsiella* bacteria were taking over my respiratory system, which frightened me. These bugs proliferated in immunocompromised, diabetic, or cancer-ridden hosts—*what was wrong with me?*

By now, the reader can anticipate the repetition of the pattern of my diminishing health in the face of healthcare ineptitude, complex diagnoses, hollow assurances, and declarations *I should feel fine.* Chronic fatigue syndrome (CFS) was explored and ruled out. Possible allergies were tested, with drastic adverse effects and the finding I now had developed severe allergies that I did not have before the surgery. Pharmaceuticals were used in abundance.

And nothing proved to be the "fix." I even learned the surgeon had removed normal, healthy tissue, not just the diseased segments.

Unavoidably this all took a toll on my career, and I looked for work outside the clinical setting, to minimize my exposure to multi-drug-resistant, hospital-acquired infections. With all my might I struggled on, but I did not know what I was fighting against.

Transformation

My transition to alternative medicine began when I developed epicondylitis (tennis elbow), which I could not attribute to any activity or injury.* When merely opening a door became painful, I went to a physical therapist, which helped 15 percent. I next received cortisone injections, the effectiveness of which diminished over time. Finally the orthopedist suggested surgery, stating it held only a 50 percent chance of improvement; my condition could also worsen. He offered no guarantee.

By then I knew better than to have blind faith! When a physical therapist recommended **acupuncture** (see Glossary), my immediate cynicism was tempered by my wariness about surgical outcomes. With acupuncture, I figured there would be little risk of injury, and it possibly could be helpful. I would try it.

At my first appointment, the young acupuncturist took a detailed history, looked at my tongue, checked my pulses in both wrists, and asked me to lie on a table before inserting several needles in my arms and legs. After the treatment, she asked if I was willing to take some herbs to treat my lungs. Fighting another bout of bronchitis and on the brink of pneumonia, I welcomed the

---

*   Only much later, after researching causal factors for my tennis elbow, did I realize Cipro had damaged my tendons and ligaments. Today, that class of antibiotics is required to have a black-box (FDA) warning about damage to ligaments, tendons, and organs.

suggestion. She gave me two bottles of small, brown-and-red pills and recommended a salve to rub on my chest.

To my amazement, I felt better within two days and no longer produced as much phlegm. Acupuncture and the herbs had helped my lung infection in a way conventional medicine had failed. Over time, the tendonitis improved, as well. My cynicism softened to skepticism, but I was not converted—yet.

The second catalyst along my transformation to integrative medicine occurred in 1996, after a simple comment made by Dr. Harley Haynes, the chief of dermatology at the Brigham and Women's Hospital. I knew Dr. Haynes from the VA hospital where I worked. Kind and personable, he cheerfully provided care for all the veterans who needed it.

During the question-and-answer session that concluded the conference, I hoped to learn of a new and better way to treat plantar warts. Besides having struggled with these pesky and painful skin lesions myself, relatives and friends often sought my advice on what to do about them. So I asked Dr. Haynes: "What would you do if you followed all the recommendations and the treatment failed?"

To my surprise, he answered that if he tried his best for six to nine months and the warts worsened or did not resolve, he would send the patient to the psychologist down the street, and the warts would be gone in three months.

"The psychologist down the street" was Ted Grossbart, author of *Skin Deep*, which describes how he helped many people heal from previously unresponsive conditions, including psoriasis, acne, warts, and rashes. My initial fascination multiplied when I read about immunocompromised cancer patients who had widespread warts for three years that disappeared after psychological treatment.

Why had I not learned of this in medical school, at conferences, or in the mainstream medical literature? Why wasn't this the standard of care? After reading the book, I spoke with Dr. Grossbart, who said, "The treatment is very simple. It's **hypnosis** (see Glossary), and all hypnosis is self-hypnosis. Anyone can learn it."

Well, I thought: if it worked for warts then it might work for my sinus problems and pulmonary infections. After all, warts are due to viruses, which are infectious agents.

Within two weeks I saw an unusual notice in the *New England Journal of Medicine* for a training in hypnosis. I signed up immediately. I also looked for a hypnotherapist *not* affiliated with Harvard, because I felt embarrassed to work with a colleague. At the time, I believed seeing a psychologist signaled personal weakness.

During the training, I witnessed and experienced healing in a way I never had. Hypnosis enables communication with the unconscious mind, allowing insight, learning, and transformation, which I saw demonstrated in real time with volunteer subjects. I witnessed people undergoing life-changing insights and finding peace within themselves. Moved by the experience, I began to listen to myself in a fresh way and experienced a renewed well-being. I gained tremendous respect for hypnosis and its practitioners. Subsequently, I attended the National Institute for Clinical and Behavioral Medicine Conference and volunteered to be evaluated for a demonstration on orthomolecular medicine. The speaker had no knowledge of me and yet was able to determine my medical history by evaluating me with his words and a hand-held probe applied to various points on my fingers (corresponding to meridian points in Chinese medicine). He informed me that my immune system was stressed, I had taken too many antibiotics, and my lungs and sinuses were weakened. Shocked that a stranger could determine within three minutes—with astonishing accuracy—so much about my medical history, I puzzled: "How can this be?"

Excited to explore other modalities, I attended a **Qi Gong** (see Glossary) workshop on breathing, by Kenneth Cohen, a Qi Gong master. After talking about the dynamics of respiration, he guided us through several practices. For the first time in many years, I enjoyed a deep, satisfying relaxation. Moreover, what I learned about breathing and its effects on lung function and well-being has delivered lifelong benefits. Breathing is so much more than just a necessity for life. My breathing rate decreased to five times a minute, my heart rate (normally in the seventies) went down to fifty. I was thoroughly relaxed. A slower respiratory rate and a slower heart rate denote a deep state of relaxation and well-being (when there are no symptoms of distress or weakness).

Next I went to a **Focusing** (see Glossary) workshop, where I learned a new way of listening, i.e., being present with feelings, mine and others', and noticing without judgment. This practice reduces stress and increases insightful understanding of situations and emotions. I felt comfortable with Focusing, since scientific evidence supported its effectiveness for relaxation and health in breast cancer survivors.

Energized and feeling renewed optimism, I was determined to explore and master these skills and practices. As if traveling in a foreign country, I began to learn the language, customs, and laws. Under the guidance of a psychologist experienced in Focusing, I signed up for a training. At first I learned the method as a self-directed process, with the therapist *holding the space* and asking questions that allowed the subconscious to explore possibilities for healing. Later I became a Focusing trainer.

More wonders awaited. In a workshop on **Healing Touch**, taught by students of Dora Kunz, RN, I watched as two nurses used their hands to scan a volunteer. They noticed a void in her chest behind her heart, and she revealed she had been operated on for esophageal cancer five years earlier and therefore had a missing part in her chest. This was beyond my comprehension. How could someone, just by passing a hand over the body, know about inner anatomy? I felt like a child watching a magician, except no magic, no deception existed. Moreover, this woman with esopha-geal cancer was thriving—that was unheard of in medicine. She told me she had been working with alternative practitioners and had a special diet.

I took a **Tai Qi** (see Glossary) class and committed to studying Qi Gong with Ken Cohen. I practiced Qi Gong every day, doing standing meditation and other practices to deepen my breath and sense of well-being. I consulted with an **orthomolecular** (see Glossary) physician about nutrition and supplements, eager to inte-grate these powerful treatments into my regimen. At my first visit, which lasted two and a half hours, the doctor informed me I was allergic to many foods and deficient in many vitamins and miner-als. For the next six weeks, I restricted my diet to rice, eggs, lamb, green vegetables, almonds, apples, pears, limes, some root vegetables, and dozens of supplements, vitamins, and minerals. I stopped eating most grains, dairy, cow meat, chicken, and baked goods. Within a week, I felt revitalized, and my sinus congestion seemed to resolve. Because I felt so much better, I gladly followed this limited diet. Over the next few months, my regimen became less strict; however, I still avoided various foods containing wheat, dairy, or flour.

Despite having clinically significant, infection-free periods, I still had more healing to do. Eventually, an infectious disease spe-cialist made the diagnosis of bronchiectasis, which a CAT scan confirmed. This is the same condition people with cystic fibrosis have in their lungs.**

** How on earth had I developed this? I cannot be certain. Today I believe the root cause of my infections began when a dentist insisted on replacing thirteen fillings with a "new, improved amalgam." At the time, few professionals understood the extreme toxic load such treatments place on the immune system. I also suspect complications from surgery exacerbated my ailment, since my problems worsened after the second operation. I had been intubated, and my airway may have been unprotected coming out of anesthesia.

Standard treatment involves cycling antibiotics or taking antibiotics every other month. A genetic predisposition to cystic fibrosis was also ruled out. With the support of my internist, infectious disease specialist, and alternative health providers in homeopathy, acupuncture, functional medicine, and **energy psychology** (see Glossary), I learned to manage my bronchiectasis. I resorted less often to antibiotics, and when I did take them, I did not need to take them as long. Herbs and nutrition supported my immune system and my lungs.

Over the past ten years, I have resorted to antibiotics only four times. Whenever I did, they were effective in abating the infection but still left me weakened. However, working with my teachers and colleagues, the intensity and duration of each bout shortened with energy psychology and sessions in energy healing like **Reiki, Reconnective Healing,** and **acupuncture** (see Glossary). My lung condition remains stable as I follow the principles and practices I learned, and I feel much healthier and able to enjoy life again.

Discussion

How and why does a well-educated person keep expecting success from the same medical treatments that repeatedly failed? I don't know all the reasons; following are some that come to mind.

The dogma of modern education and science. My education—grounded in science, facts of physiology, anatomy, pharmacology, and cell biology—made sense to me. Plus, I had invested several decades in learning and practicing what I believed to be solid knowledge. I was not willing to accept, and did not want to see, that the science of medicine is fallible and incomplete.

Past success. Practicing medicine had given me fulfillment and satisfaction. I had saved many lives and improved the health of thousands of people. Medicine worked and was lifesaving.

11

Following convention. As a resident, I remember a colleague who saw his patients while being attached to an IV pole for hydration, because he had a severe episode of gastroenteritis. He became the exemplar of what a doctor should be: a trouper, a good soldier who does not falter and does his share, no matter what happens. I adopted this as my definition of dedication, and I believed in being dedicated. I did the same thing; I pushed myself to maintain my normal work duties, and few realized how ill I was. Rest, for me, was out of the question.

Shame. I felt shame and guilt for being unwell. When my condition didn't heal, I blamed my body and not the treatments. If I couldn't heal myself, how could I be worthy of being a doctor? I needed to model health for my patients. How could they respect me if I was sick?

This was a perplexing factor, because it ran contrary to the way I treated others. I saw lawyers, judges, business people, teachers, plumbers, and farmers coming in with infections, heart disease, back pain, and abdominal pain. I didn't think less of *them* for being sick. Often I prescribed time off from work and recommended avoiding stress, and I felt happy to give them time to relax and get better.

Unrealistic expectations. As a resident, even when ailing, I woke up at 5:00 a.m., did aerobic exercise for forty-five minutes, and ten minutes later I was on my way to the hospital to take care of my patients. I expected my body to be strong, invincible, and resilient. I never suspected I was using up my reserves without replenishing them. Such information had not been part of my education. Bodies were systems that could be fixed with medications and surgery. Moreover, I didn't realize my body's ability to heal had been compromised by taking antibiotics, having surgery, and other stressors.

Self-sacrifice. Brought up to be considerate and to think of others' needs before my own, I believed sacrificing myself was the right thing to do, if others benefitted. I was needed, and I had to show up.

Pride. The general attitude in the hospital regarded patients as being helpless without physicians; they could not heal themselves. While I now recognize the grandiosity of this view, at the time I believed that if I didn't provide the care they needed, either they would continue to suffer—which was unconscionable to me—or someone else would be enlisted as the caregiver.

Training. Residents commonly identified patients by the diseases they had. For example: "I admitted a GI-bleed, an asthmatic, and an MI." (*GI* is the abbreviation for "gastrointestinal" and *MI* represents "myocardial infarction," or heart attack.) People became the housing for disease. Doctors treated the disease rather than the person. So admitting to being sick meant *I was the problem*, rather than I *had* a problem.

Limiting beliefs. My training in chemistry and medicine focused on science and allopathic (conventional) medicine alone. As a physician, my belief in the superiority and authenticity of Western practices reigned absolute. I had rejected older traditions and anything modern science could not prove. I had succumbed to the negative bias—perpetuated in American culture through the media and through "big pharma" advertising—that modalities such as acupuncture, homeopathy, and chiropractic were aligned with quackery and witchcraft and not worthy of consideration.

In conclusion, I share my own medical history and dissect my experiences and beliefs because I know I have much in common with others who have health challenges. I have not been alone in my quest; you needn't be, either. And like me, I hope you will be renewed with optimism and excitement about the possibilities for attaining happiness and health.

EXERCISE: FOOT MASSAGE FOR RENEWAL
10-15 minutes

You will need a lime, small lemon, or small ball of rubbery consistency for this exercise.

Stand up and walk barefoot on the floor. Notice how your feet feel; notice your breath, your arm swing, your neck, and your shoulders; notice how you feel.

Place the lime under your right foot and start rolling it. Use the sole of the foot for one minute, keeping the lime in the center of the sole.

For another minute each, roll the lime using:

- the outer side of the sole
- the inner side of the sole
- the hollow (arch) of the foot
- the outer side of the arch
- the inner side of the arch
- the center of the heel
- the inner side of the heel
- the outer side of the heel

Notice the scent.

Let go of the lime. Walk again.

Notice how you feel. How does the right side of your body compare with your left side?

Notice your breath. Does it feel the same in your right lung and in your left lung? Arms? Legs?

Repeat the exercise with your left foot.

Chapter 2: Jacob

A Case of Abdominal Pain

We look for medicine to be an orderly field of
knowledge and procedure. But it is not. . . .
There is science in what we do, yes, but also
habit, intuition, and sometimes plain old
guessing. – Atul Gawande, MD

IN THE MID 1980s, before I began studying alternative methods, I worked as an emergency physician in the Boston area. In the ER, there was only one physician in charge at a time. When my shift started at 3:00 p.m., I assumed responsibility for the patients, taking over from the physician who was leaving. Likewise, when my shift ended, I would sign over any remaining cases to the doctor succeeding me.

Being a member of the Massachusetts Emergency Physicians Association, I learned that some of the patients most likely to slip through the cracks were those who were signed over between shifts. So I always performed a comprehensive evaluation to make sure I wasn't missing anything. One memorable day, a young marine in the ER waited on the brink of that crack.

When I arrived at work, the doctor finishing his shift informed me that he was signing over one patient who had not yet been evaluated because he was considered a private patient, expecting a consult with a general surgeon. The young marine, however, had serious symptoms, including abdominal pain and vomiting, lasting over two days, without diarrhea. This raised the suspicion of a "surgical abdomen" (a condition requiring emergency surgery).

Because the surgeon had been tied up in a gallbladder operation for over two hours, the ER staff conducted blood tests and an x-ray of the abdomen, to rule out the immediate concern of an intestinal obstruction. After hearing this report, I asked the nurse to take me to the young man before checking on other ER patients. In this, I acted according to my intuition and contrary to customary procedures.

Marines are famous for their fitness and strength, but the young man I saw sat upright on the gurney, clearly distressed, incapacitated, and apprehensive. His eyes showed fatigue, as if he hadn't slept for several days. I introduced myself and greeted him by his first name. "Jacob, can you tell me how your problems began?"

Jacob sounded sad and weary: "Two days ago I woke up with a tummy ache and vomited. I saw the doctor at the base, and he told me to rest for two days. I felt better, but then today I had more pain and threw up my breakfast. I still have the pain, and I'm nauseated." I asked about other symptoms, but he denied being feverish or having other intestinal problems. He emphasized feeling weak.

"Where do you feel the pain?" I asked, and he pointed to his upper abdomen, above the navel. I began with the ABCs—airway, breathing, and circulation—of evaluation. Noticing that Jacob breathed rapidly, I listened to his lungs and heart, hearing evidence of fluid at the base of his lungs (rales) and an S3 gallop in his chest, both of which are signs of a tired heart. Before proceeding further, I asked the nurses to do an electrocardiogram (EKG) and test for oxygen in his blood. Within two minutes, it became clear Jacob had suffered a major, acute heart attack. The EKG also indicated electrical blockage of the heart and abnormal heartbeats.

We moved him to a critical care bed where his heart and blood pressure could be monitored. Checking his abdomen, I found it was normal. Nurses inserted an IV, and a chest x-ray was taken at the bedside. I started him on oxygen, nitroglycerin, and a strong diuretic (Lasix) to address his heart failure. He received aspirin and blood-thinning medication to dissolve blood clots that might be responsible for his heart attack. Jacob was also given a medication to normalize the dangerous irregularity of his heartbeat and decrease the risk of sudden death.

For the abdominal pain, which actually was due to his heart attack, I administered intravenous morphine, a very effective pain reliever that also lessens anxiety. This step was not just palliative care—pain and tension can constrict the supply of blood to the heart, a significant risk in this case. I reassured Jacob his abdomen was fine and that the treatments we provided would make him feel better as rapidly as possible.

I spent twenty to thirty minutes stabilizing Jacob, until the pain subsided entirely and his breathing slowed. I later learned this heart attack had been quite severe, damaging about half the muscle of Jacob's heart.

DISCUSSION

Jacob's preliminary test results were normal. Moreover, he was considered a private patient, scheduled to be evaluated by a surgeon. At that time in the 1980s, courtesy to the surgeon dictated that I should not evaluate or treat his private patient. So why did

I decide to examine Jacob, particularly considering my colleague had not been concerned?

An adage in medicine advises: *When you hear hoof beats, don't look for zebras. Look for horses.* It means one should look for a simple explanation, not for rare and unusual diagnoses to explain common problems. In this case, the hoof beats correlated to the abdominal pain and vomiting. Had they been the hoof beats of a horse, the problem would have been abdominal, such as gastroenteritis or appendicitis. Instead, I encountered a zebra, and the hoof beats indicated heart attack and possibly death. So I would extend the adage to say: *If you see stripes, check for zebras.* Knowing when to do so is an aspect of the art of medicine.

In addition, there is the element of my "gut feeling" that perhaps this young man not only experienced acute pain but also faced great risk. The gut feeling is the result of a combination of training, experience, and intuition. I used my knowledge as well as my "instinct" to make this critical decision.

In my opinion, intuition stems from the ability to apply the lessons of past experiences. It pertains to having a vague feeling or knowing that comes from the subconscious. When that knowing becomes conscious, then it is a skill. The art of medicine is being able to tap into the intuitive information and make it conscious. Because I paid attention to my patients, listening and observing closely, I learned both consciously and subconsciously to be aware of red flags, of things that look suspicious.

Today, as a mind-body physician, were I to have a case similar to Jacob's, I would use many of the same interventions, but I also would employ some of the integrative modalities I practice, to help decrease the inflammatory response by summoning Jacob's innate powers of healing. Natural healing processes exist within the body and mind of each person, though sometimes contemporary medicine and interventions interfere with them.

Finally, I would put such a patient on an anti-inflammatory diet (see Appendix A). I believe this could be the difference between life and death. You will learn more about this critical component of health as you read on.

EXERCISE: BREATHING
3-10 minutes (This exercise is not recommended for people during a medical emergency.)

Watching Jacob breathe was the first clue to his physical distress. When you are stressed, breathing is shallow and uneven; however, when you intentionally slow down your breath, your body responds accordingly.

Just as your emotions, such as pain and fear, can affect the way you breathe, intentionally controlling and slowing down your breath can influence your physical and emotional experience.

Sit comfortably with your eyes open or closed.

Notice your natural breath. Is it open and free, or constricted?

Now inhale to the slow count of 4.

Hold your breath to the count of 4.

Breathe out to the count of 4.

Hold your breath to the count of 4.

Repeat for 3-10 minutes.

Notice how you feel after the exercise.

Notice your natural breath.

How has it changed?

Chapter 3: Tim

A Case of Hiccups

To study the phenomena of disease without
books is to sail an uncharted sea, while to
study books without patients is not to go to
sea at all. – William Osler, MD

IN THE LATE 1980s I worked as the first emergency physician at the West Roxbury VA Hospital (Veteran's Administration), where only veterans received services. Nights were often quiet, with only a handful of patients, while the days were busier, when about twenty to forty veterans presented for evaluation and treatment.

One Friday morning, I walked into the ER and was informed by the nurse that the night had been uneventful. One person remained. He presented at 5:00 a.m., hiccupping so continuously that he couldn't sleep. The nurse grinned and said, "His wife wanted to drop him off for the weekend." Her comment referred to the fact that homeless veterans would sometimes come for dubious medical reasons, hoping to be admitted for a few nights.

The statement felt unkind to me, and more importantly it didn't make sense: this veteran had a home, a bed, and a wife. Why would he come to the ER at 5:00 a.m.? Additionally, his chart was more than an inch thick, indicating real health problems. The nurses had taken his vital signs (blood pressure, heart rate, and respiratory rate) and assessed that he was stable and could wait until I arrived for treatment.

I walked over to the patient's bed, greeted him by name, and introduced myself. Tim was a large, fifty-year-old, stocky man who looked tired. I asked the usual question: "Will you tell me what brings you here?"

He said he awoke with the hiccups about 3:00 a.m. They wouldn't stop no matter what he tried, even though he did everything possible, including putting his face in ice and holding his breath.

He looked uncomfortable and ill as he spoke, yet as I observed him and paid attention to the hiccups, I did not feel substantially impressed by the intensity of the hiccups or their apparent effect on him. I proceeded to do a review of systems. This part of taking a history explores general questions about symptoms such as headaches, pain, malaise, rashes, and organ problems, like lung and bowel.

Tim said, "I don't feel well, Doc. I have just a bit of a headache. It's been there for awhile."

I explored this vague complaint further. He reported no chest pain, nausea, or vomiting. However, he had not been eating, chiefly because he lacked an appetite. Continuing the physical exam, I checked his eyes, ears, nose, and throat. I listened to his lungs and heart. I felt his abdomen, his arms and legs, his pulses.

Then I did a complete neurological workup, though this was not a normal procedure for hiccups. Tim could not remember the date. He was right-handed, but he seemed weaker on his right side. When I tested his reflexes, his right big toe moved in an atypical manner—a positive Babinsky, a finding that indicates a brain problem.

Though he was a strong man who could resist with any muscle I tested, I checked to see if he had a pronator drift. This is a very sensitive test for arm strength and weakness. Indeed, he exhibited a pronator drift on the right side. He also had slightly hyperactive reflexes on the right.

Seeing hard evidence of a left-sided neurological problem, I requested an emergency CT scan of his head. I ordered an EKG and blood tests and instructed that he be monitored and have intravenous access.

The CT scan revealed a subdural hematoma—bleeding in the head—on the left side of his brain. This life-threatening condition explained his weaker right side, his headache, nausea, and possibly the hiccups.

DISCUSSION

Hiccups are a relatively common and typically benign occurrence, usually self-limiting, and rarely require medical intervention. When they persist (more than forty-eight hours) or prevent comfort and sleep, textbooks or medical trainings recommend prescribing an antipsychotic medication, such as Thorazine, which often is effective in stopping them.

Hiccups are generally considered to be the result of spasms of the muscle separating the chest from the abdomen (the respiratory diaphragm) and the muscles that move the ribs as we breathe (intercostal muscles). The etiology of these spasms is poorly understood and may be attributed to metabolic, anatomic, or physiological conditions affecting the brain, abdomen, or chest.

So what compelled me to do a detailed neurological exam for someone showing up with a few hours of hiccups? What kept me from discharging him with a drug to stop his hiccups? In evaluating this veteran, I regarded him as a courageous man who only would come to an emergency room for a significant purpose, even if it did not appear serious. Most veterans come for critical or acute problems. Yes, some present to the ER because they can't otherwise get a quick appointment, but to show up at 5:00 a.m.—an inconvenient hour—is not typical. For me, this was a subconscious red flag, a flag that may very well have saved Tim's life.

In retrospect, there were other red flags that directed me to do the neurological evaluation and examination of this man as if he had intractable hiccups (lasting a month or longer), rather than hiccups of a few hours:

- The diaphragm is a breathing muscle. What controls this breathing muscle? The brain.

- The patient said he did not eat and was not hungry. For a large man, this is unusual. Nausea can be from the stomach, but it also can be from the brain.

- People who *do* eat when they have something adverse happening in the brain may be nauseated and may vomit. Was that why Tim was not eating?

Some doctors might have felt I spent too much time evaluating patients. The time I spent with Tim was less than twenty minutes, with most of it devoted to listening and observing; the exam itself took less than ten minutes. Checking for a pronator drift is a simple, sensitive diagnostic test that can reveal subtle but significant findings. It consists merely of asking him to raise both arms, with the palms facing the ceiling, and close his eyes. Even a slight weakness will cause an arm to turn inward.

This is what I mean by the *art* of medicine: listening to what is *not* said, looking for relevant signs, seeing the big picture, and treating all patients as though everything they say matters. It has to do with knowing the science and using it to solve the puzzle. Often some pieces of the puzzle are missing, so you have to use your knowledge and your intuitive mind. This is also the basis for mind-body medicine—both for the professional and the patient. Sometimes the brain knows subconsciously and can provide what the body needs for healing.

EXERCISE: FELT SENSE
5-15 minutes

A "felt sense" (see Glossary) is a subtle bodily sensation elicited by a thought, experience, or action that is specific for that experience or action. It conveys subconscious meaning and information. It was defined by Gene Gendlin and is often a key to resolving problems.

Part I

Allow yourself to feel comfortable. Sitting still, notice your breath. Think of something that annoys you: a person, situation, or event. Notice how it feels to be in the presence of this person, situation, or event. What does it feel like?

Notice how it feels in your chest, your heart, your gut. How does it affect your body?

How does it affect your breath? Does your breathing feel shallow? Constricted?

Now let go of this situation, person, or event and return to your normal state.

Part II

Allow yourself to feel comfortable. Sitting still, notice your breath. Think of something you love dearly: a person or pet, an object, or a place in nature. Notice how it feels to be in the presence of this person, object, or space. What does it feel like?

Notice how it feels in your chest, your heart, your gut. How does it affect your body? Are you feeling more relaxed?

How does it affect your breath? Does your breathing feel deeper? More open? Stay in this state as long as you wish.

Chapter 4: Ryan and Paul

A Case of Warts

In the vastness of the ocean there is no ego.
— Deepak Chopra, MD

I HAD AN opportunity to treat two boys, brothers, because each had worsening foot lesions. Their father reported they had tried various over-the-counter medications without resolution. Initially he asked if I could prescribe an effective medication used in Canada that was not yet available in the United States. We agreed I would see his children and then let him know my recommendation after an examination.

Two days later he arrived with his sons, eight-year-old Paul and ten-year-old Ryan. The boys sat in chairs next to each other. They were neatly dressed and wore socks.

I always like to hear the story of the illness or ailment directly from the patient. To me, their perception of the problem and how it started is very informative. Ryan reported that the rash began as a small spot that he first noticed two years ago. In the previous two months, it had grown in size and caused pain when running, especially after swimming. Even walking barefoot had become painful. He stopped going to the pool, but the rash became larger and more painful. His younger brother giggled and nodded his head in agreement.

I asked them to take off their socks. Their feet looked clean. Ryan had a small dark spot about 3/16 of an inch in diameter. It had specks of black inside but had no tenderness, swelling, wetness, redness, or odor. Paul had two similar lesions—one the same size, the other smaller. They had what many people, particularly kids, get: common warts.

I asked their father if he wanted me to do energy work to help them heal the warts. He consented, and I asked the boys to close their eyes. I encouraged Paul to imagine that he could see inside his foot where the wart was and to describe it. "It's like a hole that's not too deep, with black dirt inside."

I asked him what it would sound like if it could talk. He made a face. At first he said it didn't speak, but then he yelled, "Aooowwwwwooo." He also said that it would smell like dirt.

His older brother shared a different experience. "It looks like a little blob of ice cream. It sounds like a plant growing. It smells like feet."

I set the intention for healing and asked the boys to participate in the process. They looked puzzled, but they complied. We went through a few rounds of EFT (Emotional Freedom Technique, see Glossary). This modality is performed by tapping on specific acupuncture points on the face and body, repeating key affirmations, and reciting relevant words. I guided Paul and Ryan, using their own words:

Even though I have this wart, I deeply and completely love and accept myself and all my feelings about it.

Even though I have had this wart for two years, I deeply and completely love and accept myself and all my feelings about it.

Even though I have these painful warts, I deeply accept all of myself and my warts.

Next we tapped on the acupoints and continued expressing love and acceptance for the various terms they themselves used:

This wart . . .

This speck of dirt . . .

This blob of ice cream . . .

This pain . . .

It grows like a plant . . .

It screams, Aooowwwwwwooo . . .

It smells like dirt . . .

It hurts when I walk . . .

It hurts more when I run . . .

It's been there two years . . .

I encouraged them to talk about their feelings, and then I continued with a blend of energy psychology techniques. I sensed a shift and observed the boys yawning and getting sleepy, a positive sign that the protocol was working.

At the end of the session, I asked them if they noticed any difference. They both nodded. Ryan said, "There's a weird energy going to my foot. It feels like it's healing." He also noted that the wart now looked like a yin-yang symbol and smelled like salt water. Paul just giggled and said he felt hungry. Ryan agreed.

Their father, a tennis coach, contributed his experience. During the process he had focused on a pain in his elbow that had bothered him for six months. As he participated, his elbow felt 70 percent better.

By the end of the hour, we all believed that our goal had been achieved. I recommended a specific medicated solution to apply to the warts and set an appointment for the brothers to return in four weeks. The warts were diminished in less than a month; within six weeks they were gone.

DISCUSSION

Warts are very common, frequently tenacious and difficult to eradicate. The medical literature is full of reports on how to treat them, such as using salicylic acid, liquid nitrogen, and other chemicals to burn or freeze the wart. These chemical processes often don't succeed.

From the 1960s through the 1980s and beyond, psychological and psychiatric practices had been used, succeeding where conventional medical treatments failed. Hypnosis has cured warts time after time, even in people with compromised immune systems (as with cancer patients). Yet despite the consistent favorable outcomes of hypnosis through abundant case reports and small-scale studies, medical schools do not teach it, nor is it found in medical textbooks. It is not discussed at conferences. It is not the standard of care.

I could have prescribed the anti-wart solution and let them go, but statistically, the chance of the medication working was small, considering the brothers had the warts for at least two years, the condition was worsening, and earlier medical treatments had not helped.

The techniques I used are a blend of EFT, Focusing, **Ask and Receive** (see Glossary), hypnosis, and other energy psychology techniques—though I prefer to use the term *integrative psychology*. Years ago I started using one modality at a time, and when I became more proficient, I found myself combining them, which facilitated the work and made it more fun.

EXERCISE: GRATITUDE PRACTICE FOR NATURE
5-10 minutes

Being "present" is being free of memories or future concerns—and just being. Accessing gratitude helps one to be fully present with a part of nature. It is a practice that can be extended to parts of your body, people, pets, and other aspects of your life.

Situate yourself in a place in nature; this can be real or imaginary. Notice the life surrounding you, the trees and the creatures. Notice what the trees do for the earth, for the air, for you in your life. They clean the air and provide oxygen to breathe, chlorophyll for light and energy, fruits for nourishment and health, shade for rest and protection, wood for building homes and furniture.

Notice and feel gratitude for all that you get from trees. Notice what role they play in this world. What would the world be without them? Enjoy the feelings of the tree's presence.

What else are you grateful for? You can vary this practice for anything in nature, like flowers, bees, or clouds.

Chapter 5: Rhea

A Case of Multiple Symptoms

It's only a miracle until we understand the
science. Then it's no longer a miracle—it becomes
a technology, a powerful technology. – Oprah

IN NATURE, ANIMALS know how to use herbs and fasting to help their bodies heal. Humans, though, have forgotten that and expect something manufactured to fix them. This issue crops up in my work with many individuals.

Rhea, an eighty-five-year-old woman, came to see me in my private office, seeking solutions for multiple, recent symptoms. Referred by a friend who had seen me, Rhea arrived with some idea about my practice in alternative and integrative methods— not so much *how* I work, just that she might expect relief from her problems, which affected her both physically and emotionally. She came with an open mind to new approaches.

We began with conversation. "Tell me about yourself," I invited. She described being active and enjoying a healthy life, until now. Though living alone, she socialized, participated in community affairs, and pursued her passion for reading books and discussing them with friends. I observed that she was alert, with a witty sense of humor. Her white hair was styled, and she dressed in loose-fitting clothes of vibrant colors. She carried about twenty extra pounds on her frame and told me that she did not exercise.

When she spoke of her health, her concern was clear. Her symptoms interfered with her active life; worse, they were not improving, despite receiving medical treatment. Rhea declared that she did not believe she had to accept these things just because—she gestured quotation marks in the air—"I'm old." She listed these problems:

1. Blurred vision. For several months she experienced trouble reading. Ophthalmic evaluation revealed vascular inflammation. She had received shots that seemed to help her right eye but not the left.

2. Memory difficulties. She forgot appointments, names, words, and spellings.

3. Legs. Walking had become painful, with pain in both legs.

4. Weight. She had recently gained ten pounds, and that made it more difficult to ambulate.

5. Vaginal discharge. A whitish vaginal discharge had developed about six months before; it was uncomfortable and profuse. Her primary care physician recommended over-the-counter creams, which did not result in improvement.

6. General tiredness.

Aside from the physical distress, these symptoms disrupted Rhea's lifestyle, and she worried about how they were increasing in both number and severity. The blurry vision prevented her from reading and participating in spirited discussions with her book club. Her lack of energy interfered with her busy social schedule.

Her leg pain restricted her mobility and well-being. The unpleasant vaginal discharge caused her to feel self-conscious.

"Have you experienced any other medical problems in the past?" I asked. Using her fingers, she ticked off three more conditions: (1) high blood pressure, (2) thyroid replacement therapy, and (3) high cholesterol. Her doctor had prescribed medications for each of these ailments and recently had started her on a cholesterol-lowering drug, Lipitor, for primary prevention. ("Primary prevention" is when a drug is used to prevent the onset of a disease. In the case of high cholesterol, according to Western medicine, the problem that correlated with high cholesterol is heart disease and heart attacks.)

"Let's focus on your list of current problems. When did they start?"

"Several months ago. But my doctor can find nothing specifically wrong. My blood tests all came back normal." With a wry smile, she added, "I don't care about being healthy *on paper*—I want to *feel* healthy."

Rhea's clinical symptoms suggested diabetes. Looking at her hands, I noticed slight swelling and redness around her fingernails, which told me her blood sugar might be elevated. (I had learned this from a doctor of Chinese medicine. From my traditional training, I also looked at fingernails to evaluate circulation and lung function.) "Do you like sweets?" I asked. "Tell me about your usual diet."

Rhea ate a bagel with cream cheese and fruit for breakfast; a salad or sandwich for lunch; and pasta, meats, and vegetables for dinner. She paused, and admitted, "I have a real weakness for pastries."

By this time, I had already formed an impression and thought I knew what was going on: high blood sugar could cause blurry vision, tiredness, inflammation and therefore pain, and yeast infections. I asked if she would change her diet, which could alleviate or eliminate her problems. She thought she ate rather well, especially because she included fresh fruits with some meals, but she was willing to try.

I advised the following:

- Avoid gluten and white flour: no bagels, bread, pasta, or pastries. Small quantities of organic, whole-grain Ezekiel bread (flourless, unprocessed sprouted grain, low in gluten) would be okay.

- Avoid processed foods like sugar and prepackaged foods, or modified foods containing corn syrup, trans fats, hydrogenated/partially-hydrogenated fats, diet drinks, or any ingredients she didn't recognize or understand.

- Avoid sweets, including pastries and alcohol, and limit fruits to one apple a day. Pomegranate seeds or blueberries would be fine with a meal.

- Increase vegetables, preferably local and seasonal.

- Include probiotic-rich foods and take probiotic supplements orally and vaginally.

- Drink plenty of water, at least eighty ounces a day (both because of living in the high desert and the probability of having elevated blood sugar).

- Walk for ten minutes twice a day.

- Ask her primary care provider to order an HbA1c test, to determine her mean blood-sugar level.

- Question her physician about her individual need for taking Lipitor, discussing the pros and cons of this therapy for her. I gave Rhea a recent publication that reported that primary prevention was beneficial for younger people but was detrimental for older people without documented heart disease.

• Obtain a copy of her blood tests for me to review and evaluate.

As Rhea listened carefully to these recommendations, her animated face became still. In the silence following my delivery, I could see Rhea weighing the information. Finally she said, "I think it would be too difficult for me to live on this diet."

I understood; such a change would mean giving up a lot of daily pleasures. Moreover, she wasn't certain that her diet lay at the root of her problems. I proposed that she try it for ten days, at which point we could meet again and re-evaluate the diet. But I could still see her reluctance. "Would you like to do some energy psychology before you leave today? It could make if easier for you to follow through with the recommendations."

Rhea agreed, and for the next thirty minutes we worked to clear negative emotions and resistance, using energy psychology techniques that entail a gentle tapping of specific acupuncture points on the face, hands, and head while speaking relevant statements, until the negative affect is cleared. (See the Glossary for a list and descriptions of these approaches.)

Rhea relaxed and cooperated, repeating after me these phrases while tapping:

Even though I have doubts about the effectiveness of this difficult plan, I am willing to consider it and be curious.

Even though I don't believe I can follow through with these recommendations, I deeply and completely love and accept myself and my feelings about them.

Even though this seems impossible, I am willing to give this new treatment a chance.

As we tapped on the facial acupoints, Rhea continued to repeat after me:

This seems crazy!
She wants me to do what?
I can't do this.
She wants me to go without bagels.
She wants me to go without pastries!
How can I not have my dessert?
Why should I deprive myself?
I'm eighty-five—no one tells me what to eat, or not to eat.
I wonder if I can.
I can try.
What if it helps?
What if it doesn't?
I could be curious.
I could try.
One hour at a time—
One day at a time—
I could certainly do one day.
Or two—
Or even more.

After a few rounds, Rhea reported feeling different and interested, even though she still had doubts about following the recommendations. So we continued with a few more sequences, and when she sighed, I noticed how her face relaxed and a smile appeared.

Concluding the session, I offered her water to drink and said, "How do you feel now about adopting these new diet suggestions?" With surprise on her face, she expressed confidence that she could follow the diet for ten days. She had no lingering reservations. We scheduled her next visit.

When she returned, Rhea exclaimed that she felt like a new woman. She had more energy; her leg aches disappeared, and she walked more regularly; her vaginal discharge decreased; she lost ten pounds; and she actually *enjoyed* the new diet. I shared her delight.

"Were you able to test your HbA1c?" She had—and learned it was elevated in the diabetic range, which confirmed my impression. She also, with her doctor's consent, stopped taking the Lipitor.

Rhea's renewed vitality glowed. Though she proclaimed the treatment "miraculous," I assured her it was very natural, very ordinary. When we balance our minds and bodies, health is the outcome.

Discussion

When someone who has been healthy develops several problems simultaneously, I look for a common denominator. Diabetes seemed possible in this case, given Rhea's signs, symptoms, and history, because elevated blood sugar can cause blurry vision, lack of clear thinking, and tiredness. So my primary concern was to normalize her blood sugar, which also would decrease the preponderance of yeast (which thrives on sugar), the likely basis for her vaginal discharge.

Yet it is rather uncommon for a woman in her eighties to develop diabetes over the course of a few months. What could have precipitated this condition? I considered that Rhea recently had started taking Lipitor, a medication commonly used to lower cholesterol, which also has been reported to cause hyperglycemia (elevated blood glucose), memory problems, and myopathy—a degenerative disease of muscles—which would account for the pain in her legs. The addition of Lipitor could have precipitated diabetes and caused those symptoms, as well.

In my practice, I sometimes advise people to explore with their health providers the necessity of taking a drug. In Rhea's situation, I knew that current protocols did not support the use of Lipitor for primary prevention in elderly people. Furthermore, when a patient in her mid-eighties develops adverse effects (diabetes, muscle aches, fatigue) after starting the statin drug, it is an indication for stopping it. Finally, the fact that she had no history of heart disease indicated that her cholesterol level was not a risk factor. Rhea appropriately asked her doctor whether she needed this drug, and I gave her scientific information supporting its discontinuation.

Diabetes can often be controlled by a diet designed to lower blood sugar. Asking Rhea to change her eating habits for ten days seemed like a simple suggestion, but I also understood her reluctance. She enjoyed her food choices—and medical standards even recommended those choices. So the biggest questions confronting me were how to convince her to eat *less* fruit, which she knew to be rich in vitamins and antioxidants, and how would I persuade her to give up the pastries she so enjoyed? Some people say they would rather die than live without their favorite foods.

I knew I had to make the choice easy and enjoyable, which is why I used energy psychology. By reframing the recommendations as an exciting experiment, Rhea felt eager to try it. Enthusiasm replaced her doubts, and she found creative ways to enjoy new menus. Later, as the Lipitor was discontinued, she began again to eat more fruit and other foods she enjoyed. Rhea is now ninety-two and doing well, still active, and traveling often.

Rhea's postscript

I think it's important in this day and age to take advantage of and explore new possibilities. Joalie uses many interesting approaches. Sometimes these were extraordinarily helpful. Other times I wasn't sure I understood everything and needed time to absorb it and respond. But I opened up to the experience of something new. And that keeps you feeling alive.

Exercise: Palming
10-15 minutes

Palming is a practice that relaxes the eyes and the nervous system. It allows the eyes to rest fully and completely. Closing one's eyes while asleep or in meditation, the eyes still work as one dreams. There is still light perception. So palming the eyes (covering them fully with your palms) allows the eyes to fully rest in complete darkness.

While sitting or lying down, rub your hands together vigorously as you breathe in.

When you exhale, place your hands on your closed eyes. Keep them there for 10 minutes without letting light in.

Notice your breath. Allow your inhale to reach your eyes, and relax the breath into your eyes with the exhale.

You can also check your visual acuity before and after this exercise. Some people see more sharply for a short period after this exercise.

Chapter 6: Claire

A Case of Chest Pain and Elevated Blood Pressure

The good physician treats the disease; the great physician treats the patient who has the disease. – William Osler, MD

CLAIRE, A PROFESSIONAL woman in her eighties whom I've worked with for years, typically calls when she has tried everything else, without the desired results, or she wants a second opinion. Her medical issues include a history of inferior myocardial infarction, a mild heart attack twenty years earlier with hypertension, and stable angina. She routinely sees her primary care physician (PCP), a cardiologist, and enjoys a good rapport with him. She takes a couple of prescription medications for her blood pressure and occasionally uses Valium for acute back pain or severe anxiety.

One Sunday morning she called, and I heard tension and urgency in her voice. She told me she had felt unwell for two days, and her blood pressure (BP) was elevated. Though she had slightly increased her medication, she still experienced a generalized malaise and anxiety, discomfort in her chest, and an irregular heartbeat, which her BP monitor confirmed.

A Valium had helped her sleep well the night before. She awoke and ate half a banana with her medications and vitamins with magnesium, but the ache in her chest persisted. Her heart rate remained irregular, and her BP was 165/75 with a pulse of 58. Most alarming to her was the development of pain around her waist, radiating all the way down to her feet, and her legs and feet felt ice cold—not cold to the touch, but they gave her a freezing sensation. Even cashmere leg warmers and a heating blanket couldn't warm her up.

Had I not known Claire for over twenty years, assisting her in numerous health situations, I would have insisted she call an ambulance and go the emergency department, and notify her doctor, too. But I knew her well. I recommended she try sublingual nitroglycerin to determine if it was cardiac ischemia (inadequate blood flowing to the heart). She took two. They stung under her tongue and she developed a headache but saw no immediate improvement in her symptoms. The stinging indicated the nitroglycerin was active.

Turning my attention to her innate capacities for healing, I set an intention for our work together. Next I guided her through a hypnotic relaxation, where she saw herself as an adolescent, quite happy, feeling loved and appreciated for having passed her national exams with high honors. In that contented state, I led her back to her current symptoms and asked what images came to mind.

She saw a small, white boat rocking on a lake. The rocking hit her ribs, and she felt anxiety. She could hear the sound of the boat creaking back and forth.

I asked her to hold certain points on her body and head, and I spoke to her heart and her body about releasing the anxiety, the uncertainty, and the pain. She shared her awareness that she often resisted feeling uncomfortable emotions.

Twenty minutes later, after more imagery and statements, I heard Claire sigh—indicating her relaxation. I proceeded with **Ho'oponopono** (see the exercise at the end of this chapter and also the Glossary) to help her feel acceptance and forgiveness of herself. She breathed deeper. She felt more at ease.

"The nitroglycerin might have helped, after all," she said. She now described her heart as if it had been swollen. "It's normal-sized now, but it feels bruised, as if something hit my ribs and heart."

Claire estimated her chest pain had improved 20 percent. She no longer felt as cold; her legs were 30 percent warmer. I asked her to drink some water with minerals. She felt better and took a bathroom break. When she came back, she reported feeling 70 percent warmer.

She again felt a swelling in her chest and in her heart. I guided her through more relaxation steps to find a place of peace. In this process, Claire began to verbalize some issues: She needed to write some directives for her will. She worried about troubling her children if she died and not being able to help them through it. She was upset, too, thinking about her sister-in-law, to whom Claire provided much-needed support.

After expressing these concerns, she reported a greater sense of well-being. Now her blood pressure measured 143/65, much better. Her pulse normalized. She felt comfortable, and the cold in her bones disappeared. She removed her cashmere leg warmers. I guided her through more visualization for the integration of the work we did. Claire felt well but also tired. I encouraged her to drink some water and rest.

When I checked in with Claire the next day, she continued enjoying her return to well-being. She asked me for a referral for a new cardiologist, though, because she was upset with her current cardiologist. She had called to make an appointment to be seen by him, but a nurse instead directed Claire to make an appointment for a pacemaker. She did not want a pacemaker—she just wanted to see her doctor.

I advised her to see her PCP, who was also a cardiologist, and to reconsider making an appointment with her regular cardiologist, reminding her that he had been helpful in the past. She could directly ask him questions about the nurse's recommendation. I added that, with the information I had, a pacemaker was unlikely to be helpful, and on the contrary, it might make things more problematic. She agreed to follow up with her PCP. That evaluation was perfectly normal. Her PCP adjusted her medications and advised her that she was not a candidate for a pacemaker, and there was no indication to warrant consideration of a pacemaker.

DISCUSSION

Practitioners need to listen to the person—the *whole* person— body, mind, and spirit. Two people with the same presentation or problem can require two drastically different treatments.

With Claire, given her history of heart disease, why did I take the risk of treating her on my own? My decision would have been difficult to justify based on traditional medical care. However, I often find that the more peculiar the symptoms, the less likely conventional medicine will be effective and the more likely the condition will resolve with mind-body interventions. Claire's problems did not follow any characteristic pattern of disease. My confidence in being able to help her with unconventional methods was founded on my prior, extensive experience with her and with other individuals.

When I set the intention with Claire, as I do with all those I work with, I am open to whatever needs healing, to the process, and to the transition happening in a safe and easy way. Just as a natural stream does not flow in a straight line but rather takes the path of least resistance, I open myself to moving in the direction of least resistance to arrive at wholeness. I have no agenda. I welcome any possibility that allows the person's unconscious wisdom to guide the healing. My role is to assist others in bypassing obstacles so that the health flows like a river that bends around hills, rocks, or mountains.

At the start of my session with Claire, I had no idea what would come up. Only by accessing information not consciously available to her and then addressing those concerns did she become able to release the gripping symptoms. Why did I use Ho'oponopono? I do not have a specific answer for that. Such work is not like medicine, where if the problem is strep throat, you prescribe penicillin. Choosing Ho'oponopono in this instance instead of another modality involved listening well, observing keenly, and trusting my own intuition and experience. People in general notice "heart pain" when they are angered or saddened. So when Claire spoke of physically feeling her heart being hit repeatedly, Ho'oponopono came to mind, and I trusted it would be what was needed to help the flow of the river bend around the mountain. The resolution of her symptoms indicated the effectiveness of this choice.

Exercise: Ho'oponopono
5 minutes

Ho'oponopono is about being one with the universe, like a drop of water in the ocean: the drop may not be the wave, but without it there would not be the wave or the same movement of the ocean. It is about the unity of the universe and the fact that we are connected and responsible for all that is.

Think of someone who is having a challenging time (that person can also be yourself). Bring them to mind, or you may hold their picture. Say the following:

> *I am sorry.*
>
> *Please forgive me.*
>
> *Thank you.*
>
> *I love you.*

The intention is to say this honestly and to summon genuine love. When you understand that being part of the universe means you might be responsible for this person's distress, then apologizing for your energetic part and sending them love and gratitude can be healing for both of you.

Repeat this a few times. Notice how you feel.

If you do it regularly, notice if anything with that person changes.

Chapter 7: Dr. Paul

Surgical Preparation for a Case of Urinary Obstruction

The practice of medicine is an art, not a trade; a calling, not a business; a calling in which your heart will be exercised equally with your head. Often the best part of your work will have nothing to do with potions and powders. – William Osler, MD

A S A HEALTHCARE provider, I consider multiple factors that contribute to successful outcomes. Preparation is a key factor, often overlooked. That is why those seeking my help are welcomed, made comfortable, provided water to drink, and learn about my methods in a conversational way, with ample opportunity to ask questions.

In contrast, one growing trend in medicine is to perform even simple surgical treatments in health centers and hospitals rather than in a doctor's office. Because operating-room time is valuable and optimized for the greatest use, procedures are scheduled to accommodate the facility's time, not the patient's. Whenever you introduce business to medicine, you diminish the fact that the primary goal is for healing to happen. Adding business or profit jeopardizes the quality of medicine.

Consequently, patients wait in a pre-operative setting that is impersonal and sterile—often for hours—alone and cut off from others. They typically receive pre-surgical instructions to fast, stop medications, or take other measures that will facilitate the surgeon's and staff's needs. Rarely do these preparations include consideration of a person's needs beyond what is dictated by the procedure.

What is wrong with this picture? A lot: a normal tendency to feel vulnerable and to worry is exacerbated, not alleviated. More importantly, an individual's innate ability to heal—another key factor to effective results—is totally disregarded. I and an increasing number of physicians actively explore ways to incorporate in our methods more integrative approaches to achieve the best medical outcomes—that is, the restoration of health—specifically by addressing an individual's emotional outlook and their natural healing powers.

Dr. Paul is a colleague still in practice at age seventy-five and a respected member of his community. Similar to "doctors" you may see on television, he is a tall and slender, white-haired man with an open and kind expression. We had met socially and professionally and discovered we were likeminded in our points of view, including the industrialization of medicine.

I had no hesitation about consulting with him when he asked for help with severe anxiety about a procedure he was scheduled to undergo for urinary obstruction. He was not sure he could go through with it. Knowing each other, we quickly became comfortable in my office. He already knew about my alternative approaches, so we turned our attention to his medical history.

Ten years prior to our consultation, Dr. Paul had urinary obstruction due to kidney stones, which caused severe pain. The stones were removed through a urethroscope (an instrument used to penetrate and visualize the urethra). The procedure had been excruciating and left a traumatic association, compounded by the not uncommon development of tissue scarring, which required an additional, painful treatment called urethral dilatation, which stretches the urethral canal to help facilitate the flow of urine.

For the past year, his urine stream had been weak, and he had difficulty emptying his bladder. He consulted a specialist, who ruled out BPH (benign prostatic hypertrophy), which might have been a likely cause for obstruction. Since Dr. Paul took no medications that might explain the problem, the urologist presumed recurrent scarring was responsible for his symptoms. He scheduled Dr. Paul for another urethral dilatation.

Dr. Paul had no other medical problems and had been healthy most of his life, so his prognosis was good. But despite several attempts to reduce his anxiety about the upcoming procedure, he remained highly distressed by the prospect of a second dilatation. "Can you help me get through this?" he asked. I assured him I could.

We started with **centering** exercises (see Glossary), which support the individual to be fully present and grounded in the moment, releasing distractions and racing thoughts, thus allowing mind and body to rest. Achieving a calmer, harmonious state, we next set an intention, articulating out loud the outcome we desired: in this case, that Dr. Paul's urinary stream be open and normal, with ease and comfort, and that his treatment be successful.

Our work together now turned to reducing his fear and dread. Dr. Paul's experience of intense pain ten years previously lay at the root of his anxiety, so we revisited that memory to clear the trauma imprint and free him from feeling stressed when thinking about the urethral dilatation. I encouraged him to describe that experience in detail. Then, using his own words, I employed Focusing and tapping techniques as he repeated after me:

I was not prepared physically or mentally for the pain I experienced, even though I am a doctor.

I had believed my surgeon was competent, but because of my pain, terrible doubts arose.

Healing was difficult, and I blamed the surgeon for some time. I felt he could have done a better job.

Though I had an obstruction, I loved my body. I loved the health I had enjoyed, and it was scary to have that jeopardized.

Gradually, Dr. Paul progressed to where he could say that he forgave his surgeon. When we reached the point where he could recall that memory without distress, we turned our attention to the upcoming procedure. Using the same techniques, going over all the possible complications, we cleared his anxiety about each one.

Dr. Paul decided to go ahead with the urethral dilatation under local anesthesia. To prepare him for a beneficial experience, we discussed what outcomes he desired, and we created a list of goals and statements to be read aloud by the surgeon and others of the healthcare team at the beginning, during, and at the end of the surgery. Such statements facilitate both the removal of emotional obstacles and the activation of the patient's innate powers to heal. (More about these statements is explained in this chapter's Discussion.) At this point, Dr. Paul felt at peace as I read these statements several times to him, fine-tuning them with every repetition until they reflected the desired experience and all the desired outcomes.

Dr. Paul's healing statements were to be stated by the surgeon, anesthesiologist, or assistant at the beginning of the procedure and repeated three times:

Dr. Paul, during this urethral dilatation, you will be comfortable and relaxed. You will be at peace, and the procaine anesthesia will keep you comfortable and free of pain. We are working as a team, and we will take excellent care of you.

To be read by the surgeon or anesthesiologist during the operation, ten minutes after the start, and repeated at twenty-minute intervals:

Everything is going very well. We are dilating your urethral opening. We are doing it in the gentlest way possible. Your body is relaxed and is already starting to heal. Your body is cooperating, and you will be fine.

To be repeated by the doctor or nurses three times at the end of the procedure:

We are very pleased the dilatation has gone well and has been successful. You will not have pain or discomfort. You will feel good and alert and will need little pain medication. You will heal quickly and easily, without bleeding or any other problems. Your body knows how to heal thoroughly and will do so safely and will get better every day. You will urinate naturally and completely, with ease and comfort.

Three days after his visit with me, Dr. Paul went for the scheduled treatment. The urologist briefly examined Dr. Paul and said that he could not perform the procedure under local anesthesia and would have to schedule a more complicated operation, using a large, rigid scope, under general anesthesia. Dr. Paul returned home, extremely upset.

Yet, to his relief and delight, when he next urinated, his stream flowed normally, and he had no more symptoms! Evidently his body had healed itself.

Dr. Paul remained symptom-free for the next four years before developing acute urinary obstruction, due to a kidney stone. He went to the emergency room and underwent the operation under general anesthesia, without anxiety or difficulties. He has been well ever since.

Discussion

What is the explanation for this amazing, spontaneous resolution? Dr. Paul and I both believe that the work we did relieved his symptoms and restored normal urethral function. I cannot offer scientific proof, but it remains a fact that this is what occurred.

In my experience, I have seen this happen in cases of cancer and migraine, as well. Many people understand intuitively—both physicians and lay people—that memories can be anchored to parts of our bodies. There exists a mind-body connection such that healing one side of the equation naturally brings healing to the other, which is the essence of traditional Chinese medicine and other indigenous modalities.

Brendt Baum, the founder of Holographic Memory Resolution®, recounts a situation during a reflexology treatment he received from a prominent practitioner in Japan. When she pressed on a specific point on his foot, he screamed. She then asked him if he had a near-fatal lung infection at the age of two and a half. He was shocked by her accuracy, as only he and his mother were aware of that fact.

While surprising, the unblocking of scarred tissue using mind-body work—such as hypnosis, energy medicine, and energy psychology—is not uncommon. In his book, *Brief Therapy, Myths, Methods and Metaphors* (Zeig and Gilligan 1990), Gilligan reports the case of a thirty-six-year-old woman who came to him with severe anxiety regarding a surgery scheduled to open her blocked and scarred fallopian tubes, so that she might conceive and become pregnant. She received several hypnosis sessions to reduce her anxiety, and on the day of the procedure, the surgeon reevaluated her tubes and found them to be open and functional. The operation was canceled, and she conceived three years later.

In my opinion, mental and emotional preparation is important for any surgery. When the protocol is performed by a caring person who reassures the patient—who in turn can trust and feel confident about a positive outcome—the success rate is much higher. Spoken intentions also benefit the surgeon and the operating-room staff.

Setting an intention and validation of the process is like saying a prayer. Repeating it and following the protocol when the patient is anesthetized gives hypnotic suggestions when the person is in a receptive state. This affects a faster, more complete healing because the patient's innate power to heal is active.

This method was popularized by a Boston therapist and Harvard Divinity School graduate, Peggy Huddleston, MTS, in her book *Prepare for Surgery and Heal Faster; a Guide to Mind-Body Techniques*. In the foreword, well-known surgeon, author, and past president of the American Holistic Medical Association Christiane Northrop states, "The guidance in this book [is to] be given out to every pre-operative patient as routinely as the operative consent form and postoperative instructions."

I have used this technique numerous times. It helps anxious patients deal with pain, trauma, and surgery. I have witnessed its beneficial effects, and I have experienced it firsthand: In 2014 I needed an operation to remove a small tumor in my neck, close to nerves and important blood vessels. I looked for a highly skilled surgeon willing to do the procedure under local anesthesia. Dr.

Michael Yee at UCLA agreed to do so and also consented to use the statements I had written for the operation. Twenty minutes before the surgery, Dr. Yee confessed being anxious about using only local anesthesia. Usually he administered general anesthesia to paralyze the patient—an important safety measure in operations where inadvertent movements by the patient could lead to poor outcomes.

In the operating room, as Dr. Yee read the statements, I could sense his anxiety. But as he continued to read, he relaxed. The anesthetist held my hand, giving it a gentle squeeze, as she repeated the statements. Dr. Yee kept me informed of each step in locating the tumor, speaking to me as he performed the surgery.

When he read the final statement, I could hear his joy as he declared this was his fastest time in locating a tumor and his shortest for completing the operation. The operating staff, equally happy, congratulated me for being such a good patient. The process held one more significant advantage: Dr. Yee knew right away that I could speak normally and that the recurrent laryngeal nerve—essential to speech and breathing—was safe. I flew home the next day and recovered rapidly, with minimal need for over-the-counter pain medication.

Surgical experiences like Dr. Paul's, Dr. Gilligan's patient, and mine support the fact that hypnosis, energy psychology, and other alternative modalities are reasonable and successful methods of healing. They may not always supplant the need for surgery, but they can consistently complement and improve medical outcomes. Surgeons can efficiently perform the most complex or simplest operation, but they cannot make the tissue that has been cut and sewn together heal and become normal again. Only when patients activate their own innate ability to heal the injured tissue, is the full measure of recovery achieved.

EXERCISE: BREATHING AND TOTAL BODY
RELAXATION
10-25 minutes

*This exercise is done lying-down, as a meditation on the breath and on moving the life energy. Practicing this exercise helps achieve an alpha-theta brainwave state with improved **heart rate variability** (HRV; see the Glossary). The greater the HRV, the healthier and more resilient the person is.*

Lie down on your back. Close your eyes. Turn your attention to your breath.

As you breathe in, allow your breath to slow down and become easy, comfortable, and long. Notice the air move from your nostrils to your lungs to your inner being; notice it expanding. As you exhale, allow your body to relax. Repeat this a few times.

With your next inhale, allow yourself to feel the breath move from your nostrils to the point between your eyebrows. As you exhale, allow the breath to release from the midpoint between your eyebrows and out through your nostrils. Repeat this a few times.

Next as you inhale, allow yourself to feel the breath entering through the soles of your feet and moving up your through your legs, belly, gut, and chest, continuing up to your shoulders, neck, and face, to the middle of the eyebrows. When you exhale, release the breath, moving from the middle of the eyebrows through the face, neck, shoulders, trunk, arms, legs, and out through your hands and feet, as if a wave were washing your body. Repeat this for ten minutes or longer.

Return to your normal breathing. Notice how you feel and how your breath has changed.

Chapter 8: Brian (I)

A Case of Anxiety

*Key elements for survival in the medical
profession would seem intuitively to be a tolerance
for uncertainty and a curiosity of the unknown.*
— Arabella L. Simpkin and Richard M. Schwartstein, MD

BRIAN IS AN energetic, sixty-year-old mental health professional in New York City. He had conducted a flourishing
therapy practice from the same office for twenty years when his
close friend and landlord died. The new owner planned massive
renovations that required Brian to find new office space. Though
the new landlord offered generous incentives to expedite the relocation, Brian couldn't even bring himself to begin the search. The
prospect filled him with anxiety.

When he called me for help, he said this anxiety interfered
with his life, happiness, and well-being. I asked him to put his
worries into words, and he enumerated several:

"The move will be difficult."

"A new place will be more expensive."

"I won't be able to stay in midtown."

"I won't have the views I enjoy so much in this office."

"I need to feel at peace and comfortable with this move. Can you help me?"

I was confident that I could. Working by phone instead of in person makes little difference for me. I am able to feel the energetic shifts, even long-distance. I asked him to describe what he liked about his current office.

He mentioned his enjoyment of the artwork and décor, the view from the window, and sitting at his desk felt as comfortable as being at home. He felt attached to the space, the building, the neighborhood, his colleagues, the prior owner, and the garden. His description seemed like that of a person he loved dearly.

I asked him to take a deep, cleansing breath and momentarily let go of his concerns. I guided him to a quiet, peaceful place and a time when he felt safety and comfort. At first he chose a familiar beach on a bright, sunny day. But then he saw a dark cloud hovering over his head that followed wherever he went. The cloud got larger as worries about leaving his office intruded on his concentration.

"How does your body feel?" I asked.

"My stomach is tight, and I'm filled with anxiety. It's a familiar feeling."

"How young were you the first time you felt this same anxiety and tightness?"

A memory surfaced of going hunting with his father when he was ten years old. Brian dreaded these outings but acquiesced to his father's wishes. He remembered keeping a stiff upper lip but later crying in private from the pain of his anguish. He did not like carrying a rifle or trying to kill innocent animals. He wanted to please his father, but the outing only served to make him feel disconnected and alone. Hunting was torture for him, and he vowed not to do it again.

When I asked him at this point to notice how he felt about looking for a new office, he said, "It's like I'm going hunting again with my father. I'm out of my comfort zone. I don't want to move, but I have no choice. I'm afraid."

Guiding Brian through the standard EFT protocol, I constructed affirmations from some of his statements and sentiments, and he repeated after me:

Even though I love my office and I don't want to move, I completely love and accept myself and all my feelings about it.

Even though I am anxious and afraid that I can't find a new office that I will like, I completely love and accept myself.

Even though I am anxious and afraid that I can't find a new office that I will be able to afford, I completely love and accept myself.

As we tapped on the various acupoints, we went through a few variations, going back and forth between his childhood hunting experience and his search for a new office:

I love my office.
I hated going hunting.
It's not fair.
How can I leave my second home?
I have to go hunting for an office.
I don't want to go hunting.

As we advanced through the process, Brian realized that he falsely assumed he would not be able to find a suitable office, although he had barely begun the search. We moved to increasingly positive statements:

I know what I like.
I know what I need.
I may be open to finding a new office.
What if I have to let go of the old one first?

This led to another memory, and he recalled finding his co-op apartment and a vacation home, despite New York's tough real estate markets. He had found those searches easy and was happy with the results. We worked on his attachment to his present office and letting go:

I wonder if it can be easy.

Maybe I can find a good place, like when I found my dream house.

Maybe I can find a good place near a park, one more spacious, one more affordable.

I am open to possibilities.

When we stopped the tapping protocol, Brian sighed, saying that it was very helpful to make the connection between his current anxiety and his experience as a ten-year-old. He understood that, on a subconscious, emotional level, he had equated his "hunt" for a new office with the trauma of hunting with his father. He also realized his difficulty in finding a new space occurred in part because he wanted to feel that he "belonged." We continued to focus on this connection and his emotions. He gradually became quiet and relaxed.

Although he still had some concerns about finding a suitable new space, Brian felt far less anxious and more optimistic about the endeavor. Over the next two weeks, he visited several offices and initially felt discouraged, as they did not meet his expectations. However, a colleague informed him of a vacancy in her office complex, in a more desirable location. It was perfect: more spacious, affordable, with a beautiful view, and it even had a doorman. Delighted with the new arrangement, Brian's concerns resolved.

DISCUSSION

Sometimes things are not what they seem. Accepting incompleteness and uncertainty—and moving on—is important in medicine and in life. Brian, of course, knew this intellectually, but he could not move forward emotionally. Fixated on the surface of his situation, he was blind to the underlying issues that needed to be addressed.

Often something residing deep in the psyche—experiences and limiting beliefs that produce feelings of fear, anxiety, resentment, and guilt—may powerfully influence our actions. A disconnect occurs between body and mind. This is distinctly apparent in people with phobias. Someone with a phobic fear of lizards, for example, may not be able to stop themselves from running away at the sight of one, despite knowing rationally that the lizard is unlikely to cause harm.

In Brian's case, his rational mind told him that he could find a suitable place, that the new owner was accommodating and offering incentives, and that he had not yet investigated available offices in desirable areas or asked his many friends and colleagues for leads. Nevertheless he panicked, because something about the situation provoked a traumatic childhood memory in his subconscious.

I could not have known that searching for an office triggered the painful experience of going hunting with his father. However, I believed that accessing the same angst in Brian's childhood would likely reveal the reason behind his resistance. I helped him bring that memory to consciousness, first by identifying his current physical sensation and then linking that to the physical sensations of the memory.

With awareness of both the present and the past, Brian could see he was not in the same situation: no innocent animals were endangered, and "hunting" for an office was a benign, helpful, and reasonable action. Moreover, he realized that he could ask for what he wanted and seek it. It was not a *hunt*; it was a *search*. Once Brian dissociated the traumatic memory from his current situation, he could be congruent in his thoughts and actions—and therefore open to possibilities around him.

EXERCISE: DREAM WORK
10-20 minutes

Dreams can be messages from the subconscious, alerting us to situations, possibilities, or concerns. Sometimes they are metaphors for something happening in life; other times they reflect an inner knowing about conflicts and fears; occasionally they may seem prophetic. This exercise is one way to be present with your dream and access insights about its meaning.

Keep a dream journal. When you wake up and recall a dream, sit with the feelings of the dream. Start writing what you remember, and notice your feelings during the dream. Notice how you now feel about the dream: where and how do you sense it in your body? (This is "felt sense"; see Glossary.)

It's okay if you don't remember details. Stay with the feelings.

Now go into the **fronto-occipital hold** (see Glossary and diagram in Appendix B) while you think about the dream. You can also use Ask and Receive to understand the message of the dream. For example:

1. *There is a part of my being that already knows what the dream's "felt sense" is telling me and what I need to learn and do.*

2. *That part of my being is willing to inform the rest of me now.*

3. *It's doing so now with grace and ease.*

4. *My mind, body, and spirit are receiving this information now.*

5. *Information transfer is now complete.*

Take a deep breath. Notice how you feel now about the dream. Notice any insights that arose. Write these in your journal.

Chapter 9: Brian (II)

A Case of Shoulder Pain

Unpredictable patient responses to treatment
. . . are far from binary. – Arabella L. Simpkin
and Richard M. Schwartstein, MD

HEALTH PRACTITIONERS TOO often seek yes-or-no answers, disregarding the reality that a spectrum of symptoms, disease, and wellness exists for each individual.

A few months after Brian found his new office, he called me again because of persistent shoulder pain. He had strained his muscles carrying several heavy shopping bags in one hand up a flight of stairs. That injury worsened over the ensuing weeks. His doctor prescribed NSAIDs (nonsteroidal anti-inflammatory drugs) and physical therapy, but his condition worsened, and he replaced the physical therapy with massages, which provided temporary relief. Although he did not stop exercising, the pain kept him from completing his usual routine, including twenty repetitions of at least two yoga moves, several pull-ups holding on to a bar, lifting weights, and bicycling. Brian became distressed, afraid that his shoulder would never improve and that he would atrophy like an old man. "I think I'm going to need surgery," he said, "as one of my friends did in this situation."

To determine his current range of motion, I asked him to raise his arm, and he reported that he could not raise it above his shoulder. Reaching up vertically was too painful. Nor could he reach behind his back and touch the lower part of his shoulder blade. Brian estimated the pain at a level four on a scale of one to ten.

We proceeded to set an intention for the healing. I guided Brian to a place of comfort and peace to get him to relax. As he visualized Fire Island, his breath slowed and deepened. He envisioned himself as a younger man, watching the seagulls on a pleasant summer day.

I asked him to bring his attention to his shoulder, as if seeing it from the outside. He described a Pinocchio-like, wooden doll's arm: well-crafted, shellacked and smooth, except at the joints where the arm looked raw. He could see the grain of the wood at the wrist and shoulder and described them as sharp and dry, as if they hadn't been perfectly sanded.

"What emotions do you feel?" I asked.

"Fear and sadness."

Moving forward with the relaxation techniques, Brian reported feeling a little better, but he still experienced the same 4/10 level of pain when trying to reach behind his back. We worked through a couple of rounds of EFT, focusing on the pain, the frustration, the limitation of movement, his inability to work out at the gym, and his fear:

Even though I have this pain in my shoulder, I deeply and completely love and accept myself and all my feelings about it.

Even though I've had this pain for three months, I deeply and completely love and accept myself and all my feelings about it.

Even though I'm afraid to lose my strength and waste away like an old man, I deeply and completely love and accept myself and all my feelings about it.

As before, we worked through a series of negative thoughts to more positive thoughts, accompanied by tapping on various acupoints:

I feel pain and soreness.
My joints are rough and raw.
I'm afraid of becoming a frail, old man.
What if I didn't have this pain?
I wonder what my shoulder needs?
What if I felt free of the pain?
How would it feel to have a healthy shoulder again?

We communicated with his shoulder in various ways. At the end of the hour, Brian reported a 70 percent improvement in raising his arm above his head and a 60 percent increased ability in putting his arm behind his back. I advised the following:

1. An anti-inflammatory diet, which was a challenge for him since I limited his fruit intake to one or two servings a day, which would not satisfy his sweet tooth;

2. Boswellia, an herbal anti-inflammatory supplement;

3. Arnica, a common homeopathic remedy that helps with injuries and musculoskeletal pain; and

4. No lifting, except light things, with his elbow glued to his waist. No pull-ups. He could do bicep curls with decreased weight, again with his elbow glued to his waist.

I also recommended that he get another medical massage and make a follow-up appointment with me in a week.

In our next session, he reported his shoulder initially felt better. He had been able to do the modified exercises and felt quite happy to use his arms in the gym. He rode his bike with comfort, even taking a thirty-mile ride, following my instructions to keep his elbow by his waist to protect his shoulder. Brian maintained the anti-inflammatory diet, although it was difficult for him.

Unfortunately, he had lifted folding chairs four at a time, two in each arm, and experienced another exacerbation of the shoulder pain. He revealed that he was packing to move from his old office and that he had much work to do both physically and professionally.

I again tested his range of motion. He could raise his arm and touch his back up to waist level, but still with the 4/10 discomfort level. However, we both noticed that he could use the arm more and be more physically active with his upper body.

To explore his persistent pain further, we set the intention for healing work, and I guided him to a place of comfort. This time he chose a brook behind his summer home, where he was surrounded by nature in dappled light, with his cat on his lap. He faced upstream, looking at the tall trees, grasses, and wildflowers. Brian wondered if this was a metaphor for trying to reach something. Why was it singularly uncomfortable to try to lift anything or reach up? Was he afraid of reaching up? These were sound intellectual questions, but not helpful.

Listening attentively to his words, tone, and feelings, I guided Brian through the EFT protocol. I wanted him to focus on his emotions and bodily sensations, on his shoulder pain, on his inability to reach up, and the related anxiety.

As we continued to work on relaxation, I drew his attention back to the issues of his relocation, when he had not wanted to move. I commented that his shoulder pain had begun soon after this. Though he had found all he had wished for in an office and knew intellectually the new space was a better place, I perceived he still did not want to move. We focused on this idea as he tapped again.

He reported a slight improvement in his original pain level, down to 3/10. I asked him to focus on how his body carried this pain, how he felt about having this shoulder pain, and how young he could have been the first time he experienced a similar feeling.

Brian recalled being nineteen, the lead singer in a rock band. He was trying to earn money for the summer and hoping to be a professional musician. However, he failed and returned home feeling defeated, his hopes crushed. He remembered bursting into tears as he left his bandmate and friend. Looking back, he said he had been mourning and was "saying goodbye to my dream." He felt the same type of mourning leaving his old office and "leaving Carol."

Carol had been the owner of the building where his private office had been. When she died, her heirs sold it. Although Brian had found a better office at an affordable price, he now felt sorrow and grief about departing. He missed Carol, who had been like a mother to him.

Brian shed tears, reliving this loss. He had not realized how much he missed Carol and that his old office kept that connection with her alive. As he experienced intense grief, I guided him to speak silently to Carol as if she were present, to let her know how much he loved her, how dear she was, how he missed her, to express how he didn't want to leave the office because he felt her presence there, and he didn't want to let go of her.

After several minutes and a few sobs, Brian reported a sense that "it was okay." He felt Carol telling him that she had moved on and that he also needed to move on, that she wanted him to be happy.

I asked him to put both hands on his heart and speak to Carol. He said, "Moving doesn't change our connection. It is not tied to any one physical space." He felt relief and was more peaceful.

We concluded the session by reconfirming my recommendations from his last session. He also agreed to hire movers to do

the heavy lifting and prevent the re-injury of his shoulder, allowing it time to heal. Within a month, he was starting to do virtual
pull-ups, and within three months he had regained his strength
and full range of motion, and he resumed his ambitious exercise
routine.

DISCUSSION

In the work I do, I frequently see people resolve one issue, only to
face another. This is indicative of the spectrum of wellness and is
entirely normal. Though a caring and kind professional, Brian did
not realize how the death of a dear, elderly friend affected him. He
had been connected to her and other colleagues for twenty years
and was sad to see her—as well as that phase of his life—pass away.

Moreover, he had not mourned Carol's death. She was not a
relative, parent, or sibling, and Brian did not permit himself this
important emotional rite. Nor did he receive comfort from friends
and family, who also did not realize the depths of his loss. He himself did not suspect how deep his attachment was. Only when he
had to separate physically from the office where so many memories of her remained did his body speak, or rather scream.

Once he accessed his grief over the loss of his dear friend—and
released the pain with tears and sobs—he could heal. When that
became conscious, he was able to move on: physically by allowing
his shoulder to heal, professionally by feeling enthusiastic about
occupying a larger and more desirable office, and emotionally by
mourning his friend and shedding his pain and grief.

EXERCISE: SHOULDER RELAXATION
4-8 minutes (If you have a shoulder injury, check first with your
doctor or physical therapist.)

Notice the feelings in your shoulders. Notice how they feel when you make big circles with your arms, as if you were swimming.

Shrug your shoulders quickly, bringing them as close to your ears as you possibly can and releasing them, 100 times.

With your next inhale, bring them up again as high as you can (almost to your ears), holding the breath as long a you can. Release your shoulders as you breathe out.

Repeat 2 times. Notice how your shoulders feel. Does the feeling of making big circles with your arms change?

Chapter 10: Abby

A Case of Obesity

If ever there were a need for true primary
prevention, improving parenting skills is
the area. – Vincent Felitti, MD

IN THE 1980s, Dr. Vincent Felitti initiated and directed the
Preventive Medicine Program at Kaiser Permanente in San
Diego. He created protocols that helped morbidly obese people
achieve weight loss—up to one hundred pounds a year—using a
supplemented fasting regimen. The success of this methodology
was short lived, though, as many of his subjects dropped out and
regained the pounds.

As a scientist, he decided to study this phenomenon. Why
would people want to regain the "unhealthy weight?" Why would
they drop out of an effective program? Why would they reject the
help he provided? Felitti found that, for many people, "Obesity
was not their problem; *it was their protective solution to problems.*"

To arrive at this counterintuitive conclusion, Felitti and colleagues interviewed 286 subjects and learned something that had
been known for years by therapists: childhood trauma not only

correlates with psychological issues but also with the occurrence of obesity and other health issues. Even though this conflicted with the contemporary medical science of genetics and practices of mind over matter, Felitti proved it beyond a shadow of doubt by embarking on a landmark investigation. He and Robert Anda, MD, evaluated and studied tens of thousands of people—working and middle class—and he concluded that adverse childhood experiences (ACE) predicted dangerous health problems, including premature death. The greater the number of adverse events experienced in childhood, the higher the likelihood of disease and disability. Adverse childhood experiences are listed below; the percentage indicates the incidence of that trauma in the tested population.

Physical abuse	28%
Sexual abuse	22%
Emotional abuse	11%
Living with adult with drug or alcohol dependence	27%
Living with adults with mental illness	17%
Witnessing violence against mother or stepmother	13%
Not raised by both biological parents (divorce, orphan, adoption)	23%
Living with someone who went to prison	6%
Physical neglect	10%
Emotional neglect	15%

Table 1: Prevalence of adverse childhood experiences (ACE) (Felitti and Anda, 1998)

In other words, 28 percent of the tested population experienced physical abuse in childhood; 22 percent experienced sexual abuse; and so on.

To help understand the health implications of these numbers, the following table demonstrates the relationship between ACE and specific diseases and conditions.

ACE Score (number of categories)	Smoking	Severe obesity	Depression	Suicide	Alcoholism	Injected drug use	Chronic bronchitis/ emphysema	Heart disease
0	1.0	1.0	1.0	1.0	1.0	1.0	1.0	1.0
1	1.1	1.1	1.5	1.8	2.0	1.3	1.6	0.9
2	1.5	1.4	2.4	3.0	4.0	3.8	1.6	0.9
3	2.0	1.4	2.6	6.6	4.9	7.1	2.2	1.4
4 or more	2.2	1.6	4.6	12.2	7.4	10.3	3.9	2.2

Table 2: Risk factors for adverse childhood experiences (ACE)

(Felitti and Anda, 1998)

Notice how just one adverse childhood experience increases the prevalence of grave medical and psychological consequences, compared to none. Moreover, notice how a combination of ACE categories significantly escalates health risks. For example, a score of three doubles the likelihood of someone becoming a smoker, and the chance of alcoholism reaches almost 500 percent; the use of intravenous drugs increases over 1,000 percent for someone with a score greater or equal to four.

These dramatic results reveal the magnitude of the problem of adverse childhood experiences and their impact on well-being and mortality. Clearly, health practitioners need to pay attention to ACE and its significance and long-term effects. Yet many continue to ignore the data. Hence, Felitti called for improved parenting skills as a first line of prevention. Furthermore, awareness of these correlations can also empower people with ACE to be prepared, to make better choices, and to address in their adult lives the origins and consequences of adverse experiences.

Felitti's findings were very much on my mind when I saw Abby, a fifty-five-year-old woman seeking help to lose weight. Each time she went on a diet, she would lose some pounds but often would gain them back—and then some more. When she came to see me, she was 252 pounds and stood 4 feet 10 inches tall.

I listened to her explain her struggles with her weight, which did not seem to interfere with an active lifestyle. She worked full time in a hospital as a nurse. She had a busy social life with many friends. A divorced, single mom, she raised two sons; one resided with her and the other lived several states away.

Abby laughed freely and shared her story with emotion and passion. Her comfort foods included baked goods like Danish pastries and donuts. She did not have time to cook and often felt famished. In between errands she frequently stopped to grab a sandwich and French fries, though she consciously added salads and fruits in her daily diet. She commuted about one and a half hours each way to and from work.

"I feel stuck," she said. "Nothing I've tried has worked, and I really don't think I can live without bread or pastries."

After doing some energy-balancing exercises, Abby followed my lead, repeating sentences while tapping on various acupoints. We tapped on the side of the hand (the "karate chop" point—see the diagram in Appendix B) as she repeated after me:

Even though I eat pastries and fattening foods, I deeply and completely love and accept myself.

Immediately, Abby's eyes filled with tears; it was foreign to her to be loving to herself. I worked this awareness into our phrases:

Even though it is difficult for me to love myself, I am willing to consider it.

Even though I don't really know how to be loving and kind to myself, I am willing to try.

We continued to tap on different acupoints (see the diagram in Appendix B) as she repeated phrases after me:

It is difficult to love myself.

I love my children.

I love my family.

I love my mom.

I love my friends.

How about me?

Do I love myself?

What does it mean to love myself?

I take care of my family.

I take care of my patients.

How about me?

Who takes care of me?

Again she teared up and took a deep breath. We continued to work on self-care, on feeling safe, and on having permission to love and care for herself. We also tapped on her cravings for and addiction to sugar.

I gently moved toward bringing her attention to the feelings behind her tears. Thoughts and images of her mother surfaced. She felt she had not received love from her mother, who had always demanded the relationship be on her terms. Her mother took from Abby. Abby expressed resentment of her mother, who seemed oblivious to her daughter's needs and desire to connect in a meaningful and loving way.

Over the course of a few sessions, we continued to work on Abby's troubled relationship with her mother; this took precedence over other concerns, including losing weight. Yet Abby noticed she no longer automatically reached for a muffin or a Danish for breakfast. She had stopped grabbing a hamburger and fries before her long drive home. Instead, she waited till she arrived home and prepared a meal with vegetables, chicken, and salad. Her appetite felt satisfied more easily, and within a month she lost ten pounds.

By the end of the year she had lost thirty-two pounds; the following year, another eighteen pounds. She still needed to use her will power some of the time, primarily in social situations where a dessert table displayed enticing pastries and sweets. But overall, she did not feel deprived and continued to limit herself to smaller portions. She lost weight steadily.

Abby's success is not surprising or unique. I have had occasion to work with groups of people who want to lose weight. I led a workshop at the University of New Mexico, where participants were curious and motivated. At the beginning of the class, each reported cravings and food addictions for chocolate, ice cream, chips, cookies, and other sweets, and they described their feelings about these foods.

I distributed some of these temptations around the room and encouraged the participants to pick them up and look at them, and as they handled the packaging to notice their feelings, thoughts, and desires. Next, as they opened the packages, they cooperatively smelled them, felt them, and then tasted a very small bite, keeping it in their mouth without swallowing.

We tapped on acupoints for their feelings, thoughts, and desires. Afterward, most expressed surprise to notice a significant change in their perception of these "foods." They found the taste less enticing, and some no longer felt the need or desire to eat them at all.

A month later, at the next session, 60 percent of the participants reported lasting changes in their feelings toward food and in their choices. A thirty-six-year-old woman said she surprised her family and friends by choosing to eat blueberries instead of coffee cake. A fifty-seven-year-old nurse said she still ate ice cream, but her craving had decreased by 40 percent, and she ate less of it. One woman said she did not notice any change in her diet or cravings; however, she slept better and felt more at peace. Many shared a similar sense of contentment and acceptance.

One middle-aged man reported his disappointment after the first session, feeling he had wasted three hours and money, and he planned not to return. Why did he show up anyway?

"I went to a wedding this weekend," he said, "and usually I'm all over the dessert table. However, I realized I wasn't interested in the desserts, and I didn't even want the cake!"

The baffled look on his face was familiar to me.

"I don't get it! It's weird, but something positive must have happened, and that's why I am here today."

DISCUSSION

This man's response is a typical one, in that many with whom I work cannot consciously identify why or how they changed—they seem like their old selves, yet their behavior or their feelings are different. They puzzle:

What happened that helped me and caused this change?
Why did my addiction to sugar decrease?
Why do I emotionally feel better?

Occasionally the improvement is permanent, but more often it is temporary, until the root cause underlying the problem is addressed and the imprint of the originating cause—frequently one or more traumas or other adverse events—is cleared.

Felitti put a spotlight on childhood adverse experiences. His research conclusions should have revolutionized medicine and health programs. What he revealed to the world is nothing less than Copernicus discovering the earth revolves around the sun. I would argue it is equally transformative, expressly because it emphasizes the necessity to periodically question and re-examine the "truths" we accept as "real."

In medicine, for example, multiple sclerosis and other conditions were considered a hysterical disorder before CT scans and laboratory tests could diagnose the problem. In the 1970s and early 1980s atherosclerosis alone was thought to be responsible for heart attacks. I remember physicians and students ridiculing a senior physician who used a blood thinner in all his patients with unstable angina or a prior heart attack. A few years later, when research validated the theory of thrombosis—blood clotting in the artery—his treatment became the standard of care. Similarly, not too long ago, the American Heart Association recommended trans fats for people with heart disease. Only after studies proved a significant increase in risk and detrimental effects on blood vessels and coronaries did they change their recommendation.

One can—and I believe medical professionals do—view obesity as a disease with complications that include heart disease, diabetes, and hypertension. Treating hypertension with antihypertensive agents may lower blood pressure, but it does not bring relaxation or comfort. The techniques I use help decrease anxiety, which in turn allows the blood pressure to decrease.

There are many approaches and tools to heal from adverse life experiences. When choosing from among the options, it is important to remember that effective modalities need not include pharmaceuticals, surgery, or starvation diets. Treating the complications of ACE helps, but preventing them is the long-term solution. Ideally, social programs that eliminate or decrease ACE—such as parenting support, education, paid maternity/paternity leave—will be made available.

EXERCISE: TARZAN YELL
2-5 minutes (Do not undertake this exercise if you have a pacemaker or an implanted electronic device.)

This exercise stimulates the thymus gland (below the breast bone) for improved immune function.

Stand tall. Make a fist with each hand. Take a deep breath. As you exhale, tap on your chest and sternum, shouting forcefully: *Hhaaaaaaaaaaah* as you breathe out with your chest and your belly.

Notice your belly and back contracting, coming closer together as you exhale.

Take in another breath, and then empty your lungs, contracting your belly toward your back, as you shout: *Hhaaaaaaaaaaah* while tapping repeatedly. Repeat for 2-5 minutes.

Return to normal breathing. Notice how you feel.

Notice your breath.

Chapter 11: Carlos

A Case of Achilles Heel

The first duty of the physician is to educate
the masses not to take medicine.
— William Osler, MD

CARLOS CAME TO see me in the fall of 2009, troubled by painful inflammation of his Achilles tendon for nearly a year. While it didn't hinder his work as a financial advisor, it did threaten this twenty-nine-year-old's goal of running the Chicago marathon in less than three hours. Three months of physical therapy for his condition had helped, but the pain returned when he resumed marathon training. He couldn't sustain the timing or distances he needed to fulfill his intention. Even a regimen of nonsteroidal anti-inflammatory medications—standard medical treatment—failed to restore him to peak condition.

Slim and fit, as most marathoners are, Carlos shared his history with a sweet smile. I pictured him enjoying his run, free of the tension in the jaw and frowns common to other runners' faces. I asked him to estimate his chances of completing the marathon in less than three hours.

"The odds are stacked against me. At best, I have a twenty percent chance."

Knowing the starting position for realizing one's goals is optimism and inspiration, I first addressed his pessimism by using Focusing and the Emotional Freedom Technique (EFT) to help him be in touch with his feelings, clear negative beliefs, and forgive himself for all the reasons that he felt he could not achieve his goals. When Carlos's face lit up suddenly and he remembered his grandfather telling him, "You can always find a way," I knew this approach was working.

At the end of the session, I asked him how he felt. He reported with a winning smile that his body was ready to run, and he now felt 80 percent confident he could run in record time. "I wish the marathon were today."

Pleased with what we accomplished, I remained alert to the reality that deeper issues could emerge as obstacles to lasting improvement.

When Carlos returned for our second session, his confidence level had fallen to 50 percent—higher than when he presented but still not enough to achieve his goal. Discouraged, he described how the pain in his heel increased when he tried to run. "I'm out of shape," he said.

Though I did discuss diet and exercise with him, I knew this would not be sufficient. Why? Because Carlos already had received medical care for nine months, and the problem persisted. We would need to explore the mind-body-spirit connection. I asked him what worried him, and he shared a list of concerns:

• His Achilles tendonitis from nine months ago hadn't resolved.

• He didn't think he could outrun those people he needed to.

- He felt out of shape, and it would take a whole year to get back in shape.
- He needed to save his energy and not run at 100 percent, maybe at 95 percent, to keep the pace to the finish line.
- He'd be running uphill the last two miles and would need extra energy then.
- He had been given jersey number 1,500—not in the first wave.
- He had not finished under three hours for over a year.
- He was getting older and feared he was passing his maximal physical abilities, leaving his prime.

We addressed each of these concerns, working with a variety of approaches including hypnosis, the felt sense, Focusing, and EFT. We made steady progress, and Carlos even reported his Achilles tendonitis resolved. But he still could not run fast enough; he did not feel strong enough.

We next worked on visualizing the race. Carlos knew the terrain well. "Tell me how it feels when you see yourself leaving home to go to Chicago for the race," I said.

"I'm excited. I feel terrific."

"Now visualize landing in Chicago—what do you do?"

"I stay in town, not too far from the starting line, and I run part of the path to train and adjust my body to the change of altitude, terrain, and weather. The evening before, I eat a substantial meal to increase my energy reserves."

"Good. And the next morning, what happens?"

"The next morning I'm still excited to go to the race. I eat a healthy breakfast and go early to the starting line."

In the next few visualizations, Carlos expressed discouragement because he had to wait in the crowd. He was number 1,500 out of 35,000 participants. "I feel impatience and anxiety mounting in my gut and chest."

We started tapping on the side of the hand, the "karate chop" point (see the diagram in Appendix B), while saying:

Even though I'm number fifteen hundred and I'm stuck behind, I deeply and completely love and accept myself.

Even though I can't move fast, I deeply and completely love and accept myself.

Even though I feel impatience and anxiety in my gut and chest, I deeply and completely love and accept myself and my feelings.

We went through a few rounds on the other EFT points, expressing the negative consequences of starting at 1,500 and then exploring its significance. As the anxiety in his gut dissolved, Carlos realized with a smile that he could use the position to his advantage. "It will force me to start slow and save my energy."

We continued with imagery until he imagined reaching the seven- to eight-mile point, where new hindrances arose. Again using the felt sense and EFT, we cleared these, as well as subsequent negative beliefs:

I'm not good enough.

I can't outrun that guy in front of me.

It's tough to run up those hills.

The process allowed new insights to emerge, and Carlos realized he had not performed well since August 2008, when the Achilles tendonitis first developed. I asked him what was happening in his life at that time.

This was the period of a serious, national financial collapse, and he recalled a major reorganization at work, when he inherited some of a co-worker's clients. His speech slowed and he looked distressed. "Some of those clients are still furious. They suffered huge financial losses." Carlos had been professional and compassionate, yet he felt guilt and shame with these angry clients, even though he was not responsible for their losses—they had invested in risky assets during the crash.

We addressed each of these negative feelings until Carlos breathed several sighs of relief. When he next visualized running the marathon and approaching the finish line, Carlos expressed confidence in running the race in record time. And although the thermometer hit 92°F that humid day, Carlos completed the Chicago Marathon in two hours and fifty-five minutes—as he had hoped!

DISCUSSION

What can conventional medicine do for a young man who wants to optimize his physical capabilities? This healthy, twenty-nine-year-old athlete was in top shape, medically speaking. His tendonitis limited his long-distance running, but even when that resolved, his performance did not match his expectations or abilities. Medically, all he could do was ensure healthy nutrition, practice with caution, limit his speed, and take care to apply sound running techniques.

Achilles tendonitis is caused by inflammation and pain in the tendons of the major calf muscles. Standard medical treatments include nonsteroidal anti-inflammatory medications, such as ibuprofen and naproxen, and stopping the activity that causes the pain. These practices were only temporarily and partly beneficial. Physical therapy also failed to resolve this problem.

The name *Achilles tendon* is derived from Greek mythology. For the great warrior Achilles, his heel was his weakness and vulnerability—and therein lay a clue as to what would help Carlos. In fact, the effective treatment proved to be working with his unconscious and clearing objections in his mind that prevented him from healing and fulfilling his potential.

Conventional medical science deals with relieving symptoms without addressing the origin of the pain and swelling. This is like being in a leaky boat and removing the water from the boat, or holding a rag to block the water from filling the boat. The boat floats as long as you keep removing the water or as long as the hole remains blocked. But how about repairing the hole? This is what body-mind medicine attempts to achieve, a concept that has been scientifically validated with hypnosis as early as the 1950s and the work of Milton Erickson and others.

Using Focusing, hypnosis, and energy psychology techniques, Carlos overcame the doubts, fears, and negative beliefs holding him back. Not only did he achieve his goal in 2009, he continued to train—and six years later he set a new goal: to complete a marathon in two hours and thirty minutes.

What determines physiological limits? What makes an athlete excel and continue to improve? Certainly practice and technique are important. Extrinsic solutions, such as exercise and nutrition, help. However, the influence of one's unconscious state of mind cannot be overestimated. With mind-body medicine, the connections, the balance, and the communications between mind and body are reprogrammed. By tapping into innate healing mechanisms and the wisdom of the body, thoughts change—and with changing thoughts, the physiology changes. The ultimate solution is often intrinsic and is accessible through the subconscious thoughts and beliefs.

EXERCISE: BACK EXERCISE
7 minutes (If you have a back problem, check first with your doctor or physical therapist.)

This practice helps the spinal column align and improves the curve of the spine. The position helps stretch muscles that are often contracted and therefore tense. Notice what happens when you allow the change.

You will need a grapefruit, large orange, or a similarly soft, round object.

Lie down on your back with your knees bent and the soles of your feet on the floor. Notice how you feel and how your back feels.

Press your body down into the floor to minimize the space between the lower back and the floor so there is no hollow. Notice how that feels. Can you totally flatten your back on the floor?

Now place the grapefruit or similar soft, round object under the lower part of the sacrum, which is the lower part of the spine between the hipbones, right above the coccyx.

Relax in that pose for 5 minutes, slowing your breath.

Remove the grapefruit or ball and notice your back. What has happened? How does your back feel? How do you feel? How much can you now flatten your back?

Chapter 12: Brandon

A Case of Laryngitis

Variability is the law of life, and as no two
faces are the same, so no two bodies are alike,
and no two individuals react alike and
behave alike under the abnormal conditions
that we know as disease.
— William Osler, MD

WHEN BRANDON SCHEDULED a phone session with me, he initially said he wanted to work on a personal issue. Though he had been to a psychotherapist, it hadn't resolved and he remained dissatisfied.

However, on the morning of the appointment, he called to cancel his session. "I need to sleep more," he said. His raspy voice and flat intonation indicated tiredness. He was troubled by the persistence of a sore throat and flu-like symptoms that had lasted over six weeks, despite medical and complementary treatment, including antibiotics. I suggested we address his laryngitis over the phone, and he agreed.

Brandon is a generally healthy sixty-two-year-old man who works full time and has many social commitments. He enjoys traveling for pleasure and business. Three weeks prior to our session, his sore throat worsened to laryngitis and a cough producing green phlegm. Yet he continued to work and even traveled for business to London and California. However, not feeling his usual energetic self, he skipped pleasurable social activities and took care to eat healthily and avoid alcohol.

On his flights, Brandon noticed many passengers coughing, and he felt vulnerable to catching their illnesses. When he returned home and his symptoms seemed worse, he went to see his doctor. Flonase (a steroid inhaler to decrease inflammation) and cough drops (generic treatment to soothe a sore throat) were prescribed. He missed one day of work, rested on the weekends and evenings, and went to sleep early rather than going to concerts or plays on Broadway. He later took antibiotics for a week, which temporarily abated some of his symptoms. A week before our session, he also started taking Chinese herbs and pills a friend, an acupuncturist, had given him.

I asked Brandon to describe how he felt, right in the moment. In a hoarse voice he repeated feeling tired and wanting to sleep. The soreness in his throat made it painful to swallow. He also felt tension in his stomach. Turning to his personal issues, I asked about what was going on in his life and listened closely as he stated, "Nothing—there are no stressful events in my life."

Through visualization, I took him to a place of comfort and relaxation, a beach he had enjoyed in his youth. He saw himself at a younger age, sitting on the sand, watching the scenery on a warm, sunny afternoon. Waves gently spread on the shore. Seagulls waddled, took flight, and glided close to the water. Boats navigated the currents and made more waves, producing a soothing sound as they lapped the beach. Brandon tasted the salty air. He smelled wet driftwood. He was twenty-six years old, felt calm, and had no concerns. His stomach felt at ease, relaxed, and warm.

"Brandon, what is in the way of feeling that calm in your life right now?" I asked. He listed a few things, and when he mentioned a problem with a specific client, I noticed a shift in his tone. I asked him to tell me more about this issue.

He talked about this client being provocative; Brandon felt violated in a way he couldn't quite articulate. "It's a matter of principle," he said. "I have to honor myself."

Again asking him to focus on his sore throat, we worked on further imagery. He pictured something in his throat about the size of an apricot, bile green in color, and shaped like an upside-down pear with a thick consistency, like gelatin. It made a sound like *eeek*. It smelled of "green apples" and tasted "sour." It felt "sad."

I asked him to keep his attention on this imagery while I guided him through EFT, tapping on acupoints, and stating facts, feelings, and emotions related to the issue.

Even though I feel something foreign in my throat, I deeply and completely love and accept myself.

Even though it hurts to speak . . .

Even though my stomach is tight and tense . . .

After a few minutes, Brandon became aware his throat was not as dry and his voice was not so gruff. "There's something comforting about acknowledging what my throat feels," he said.

We continued for an hour, using **neurolinguistic programming** (or NLP; see Glossary) and energy psychology techniques. Afterward he felt much better, and his stomach relaxed. Brandon repeated, "It feels good to be acknowledged—as if my sore throat can take its place in the past, and the present can go on without it."

He sighed and reported the dryness was 80 percent better, the hoarseness 85 percent better. His voice was clearer, more alive, with more variations in tone. I felt the tension leave his face, replaced by a faint smile. He felt much better all over, no longer tired, and he was grateful.

I asked him to revisit that image of an object in his throat. The pear-shaped object had shrunk to "a shadow of its former self." It no longer said anything—it just breathed. The tart taste was "diluted" and "very mild." We finished the session by anchoring the benefits and expressing appreciation and gratitude.

A few hours later, I received a text message: Brandon, feeling healthy and normal, was taking a twenty-two-mile bike ride.

DISCUSSION

Sore throats and bronchitis often resolve on their own within a week to ten days, without the use of antibiotics. But often doctors find that two patients with the same symptoms will have different outcomes to the same treatment. What works for one doesn't work for another. I believe underlying stress can account for many of these discrepancies, and this is one of the reasons why it is important to treat the patient, not the disease.

In this case, Brandon's symptoms lasted six weeks and continued to affect him adversely, despite antibiotics, decreasing his activities, and resting. So why did he feel better within an hour of working with me—to the point of being energized and going on a long bicycle ride? What explains this amazing transformation?

I used no medication, just hypnosis, Focusing, and energy psychology to help Brandon summon his innate healing potential. Moreover, I believe our work identified the true cause of his sore throat: the stress of the provocative client, compounded by feeling unable to express his feelings. He tried to ignore his frustration with a situation he felt incapable of changing, and the stress manifested through his symptoms.

Why did this session resolve his symptoms? It is known that

stress affects the immune system and causes inflammation. It is the body's learned, unhealthy response to trying situations. Even when an agitating circumstance is no longer active or present, one's feelings about it may sustain the stress. By working to acknowledge it and then moving toward a peaceful feeling in relation to it, clarity about the situation can emerge, with new insight and relaxation. Consequently, relaxation, gratitude, and other positive feelings decrease inflammation, and resolution of the physical symptoms becomes possible. Brandon reclaimed his health that day. He carried it with him when we completed the session, and he maintained it without further sessions.

EXERCISE: FRONTO-OCCIPITAL HOLD
5-20 minutes

The body has an energetic and complex electrical system. The skin carries a negative charge except in the palms and soles. The fronto-occipital (FO) hold has been used for centuries, believed to help facilitate communications between different parts of the brain.

Choose a concern, issue, or problem you are experiencing. Sit in a comfortable position with your spine straight and buttocks well grounded in a chair or cross-legged on the floor. Place one palm on your forehead and the other on the back of your head. (See the diagram in Appendix B.) Bring your attention to your breath while also acknowledging the concern. Invite your eyelids to close.

Notice if you start to sway. If you do, allow your body to move as it chooses, in the directions it chooses. Let yourself follow the movement without resistance and without augmenting the movement. Allow it to stop on its own.

Notice how you feel. Notice how you feel about the issue or concern you concentrated on.

Chapter 13: Valerie

A Case of Lung Cancer

The natural healing force in each of us is the
greatest force in getting well.
— Hippocrates

V ALERIE IS A fifty-eight-year-old woman referred to me by
her therapist. An elegant, outgoing woman looking younger
than her age, she had been diagnosed with lung cancer one month
earlier.

In the two years prior to this diagnosis, Valerie had noticed
increasing tiredness. In the previous year, she also developed a persistent cough. Her doctor, however, was not concerned. After some
months, she consulted a new doctor, who ordered a chest x-ray
that revealed a mass. An extensive workup led to a diagnosis of
stage-4A small-cell cancer of the lung, which meant it had spread
to other areas of her chest. She underwent a left, lower-lung resec-
tion to remove a large part of the tumor. But it had spread and got
larger, and doctors informed her they would start chemotherapy

after she recovered from surgery, though they did not give her hope to survive the cancer.

"My doctor wrote me off," she tearfully told me. She also experienced pain, redness, and inflammation in her surgical wound. Short of breath, she spoke with difficulty and coughed between words. She expressed fear and said that thoughts and feelings of isolation troubled her.

I learned her chest x-ray showed multiple tumors. She was seeing an acupuncturist and planned to visit a doctor of Chinese medicine who specialized in treating cancer. She adhered to an anti-cancer ketogenic diet, which produces a state that causes the body to act as if it is in starvation mode.

Beginning by administering the SUDS scale (see Glossary), Valerie's intense fear registered as 10/10—the highest level. After setting the intention with a prayer for healing, I guided her to a place of peace and contentment. She easily went to a beach with grass and trees, heard the birds sing, felt the wind blow gently, and enjoyed the warm midday sun. Allowing herself to go in the water, she felt "free and liberated!"

Realizing she had always believed her lungs were strong, Valerie accessed a feeling of deep sadness, and tears flowed. In between sobs she sensed a "lack of love" in her life, and said, "I won't be able to sing again." She had been a professional singer before becoming a flight attendant fifteen years ago, and singing remained her passion.

I asked her to tell me about a time she felt that same sadness in her life. She remembered returning from Europe many years ago, after performing in an opera. She went to see her parents, who both had cancer and died within six weeks of each other. A few months later, her sister died of breast cancer. Sadness overwhelmed her.

Gently, I addressed her grief about the deaths of her parents and her sister. Through our work, the feelings of severe sadness and loss resolved. However, heartache and pain remained attached to the possibility (and in her own feelings, the probability) that she would not sing again.

Understanding we had reached a deeper level of grief, I guided her to access a memory from her childhood when she had felt that same sadness. She remembered being four years old, when her only joy was listening to music with her ear glued to the radio. Valerie expressed surprise to experience intense loneliness and misery looking at her four-year-old self, and she realized how unloved she felt because her mother favored her younger brother and did not seem to have enough love for all her nine children. Listening to the radio had been Valerie's main source of comfort.

Using the **Core Transformation** process (see Glossary), I guided her to recall her deepest longings when she was four. Through alternating tears and laughter, she recounted memories of being loved, laughter and joy, and having caring and loving friends. The memory of being four no longer brought her intense sadness. She integrated her four-year-old self into her being in a safe and wholesome way.

After that integration, I asked Valerie to put her attention on how her doctor "wrote her off." She said with a chuckle, "He's a jerk! Somehow I feel they're wrong—I'll prove them wrong."

Next I directed her attention to the time she returned from Europe, when both her parents and sister were dying of cancer. The memory now felt more distant, her grief less palpable.

At this juncture another sad memory surfaced in connection with the events of September 11, 2001. She agreed we had accomplished a great deal that day, and we needed another session to address the 9/11 issue in a mindful and effective way.

In closing, I gave Valerie homework to help correct her energetic balance: doing the collarbone breathing exercise (see the diagram in Appendix B) at least three times a day. I mentioned

Joanne Callahan (the wife of Roger Callahan, founder of Thought Field Therapy (TFT)), who incorporated this exercise and other alternative therapies to heal from stage-4 large-cell lymphoma, and she had been free of cancer for twelve years—a fact Valerie found comforting. I also recommended topical herbs to help heal her surgical wound, as well as a homeopathic remedy for the pain.

The after-session questionnaire revealed that the session, though difficult, helped her realize how "very, very sad I am feeling." She also stated, "I feel good."

Finally, I asked her to complete the sentence: **I am still *not* ready to _____.**

Valerie astonished herself by replying, "Get well." She had no inkling such a thought or feeling existed in her.

Next I asked her to complete the sentence: **I am certain that what I *will do* is _____.**

Valerie stated: "Get better."

Both of us noticed the contradiction. I assured her this was very helpful for me so we could address these feelings in our future work.

During the next session, we cleared more trauma around 9/11 and worked on forgiving those who had been cruel and hurtful to her. We also worked on Valerie forgiving herself.

In the third session, we worked on clearing an intense feeling of disgust she had about the lung cancer, as well as more forgiveness. I helped Valerie get in touch with the part of her that felt afraid of living and wanted to die. We worked on clearing these feelings, and by the end of the session she had no desire to die and wanted to live fully.

She again found the session difficult, but learning about Ho'oponopono (see Glossary) helped noticeably. She realized she wanted to visit a dear friend and to laugh more. "I'm going to watch something funny. It's really important to laugh."

In subsequent sessions, she cried and laughed, releasing hurts and grief. We worked with imagery, and she visualized her lungs being pink and clean, with healed scars and no toxicity. Memories that had distressed her no longer brought pain or suffering. She felt more at peace, more alive, and more buoyant. We continued to work on the feelings of lack and not feeling "enough."

Six weeks later, in our last session, Valerie was singing again and also taking dancing lessons. Her oncologist informed her there was evidence of scarring where the tumor had been and no evidence of tumor progression. Five months later, Valerie resumed working as a flight attendant and was doing well, making time for singing and dancing in her life. Eighteen months later, she remains healthy and continues her wellness therapy with my colleague.

Discussion

Valerie's story is a dramatic one of overcoming a challenge and finding an opportunity to grow and heal. As a conventional physician, I grasped her oncologist's understanding—or rather, misunderstanding—of her situation. He "wrote her off" based on the scientific beliefs of her condition, something I had done with a patient thirty years earlier.

The patient I saw then presented with vomiting and dizziness. Upon examination, I discovered he had nystagmus, a movement of the eyes that causes vertigo, whose underlying cause is commonly a viral infection of the inner ear. However, this gentleman exhibited other signs of neurologic dysfunction. An emergency CT scan confirmed he had several tumors in the brain.

His medical prognosis was imminent death, but at first I only informed him of the findings. Understanding the seriousness of the situation, he remained calm when he asked me how long he had to live.

I replied that no one could tell. I did not want to be the one to tell him. But he insisted on a time frame, and I said, "six months," when actually I was thinking *six weeks*.

Had I known then what I know now, I would have informed him of possibilities for healing, knowing he risked nothing since the best conventional medical treatment could not give him hope.

Valerie received the benefit of both her therapist's and my new knowledge. However, she chose not to share her therapeutic experiences with her oncologist. This is not uncommon. Others, even professionals, make the same choice. In his book *Let Magic Happen: Adventures in Healing with a Holistic Radiologist*, Dr. Larry Burk reports on a South Carolina businessman, Norman Arnold, diagnosed with pancreatic cancer metastatic to the liver and lymph nodes.

The prognosis for such a condition is dismal, with no hope of survival. Mr. Arnold sought the help of holistic and alternative practitioners, followed a strict macrobiotic diet, and radically changed his lifestyle. He also participated in an experimental research study using mouse monoclonal antibodies (substances made in a lab to assist a person's immune system to fight cancer), but he did not inform the investigators of his other treatments and dietary changes. There were 250 participants with metastatic cancer. Mr. Arnold was the only survivor and remained cancer free ten years after the diagnosis.

VALERIE'S POSTSCRIPT

A year and a half later, Valerie is on a whole-food vegetarian diet. She has remained free of cancer. After the one-year assessment of her cancer, Valerie wrote to me: "My oncologist is bound and determined to find more cancer in me, so she ordered a brain scan and another PET scan. But I'm bound and determined to disappoint her again. Ha ha."

She also gave me permission to share her answers to a questionnaire I regularly use with clients:

CLIENT QUESTIONNAIRE

What brought you to consult with Dr. Joalie Davie?

I was diagnosed with stage-4 lung cancer and was terrified. My therapist recommended I talk to Dr. Joalie Davie. I didn't really know what to expect, but at that point I had nothing to lose.

What did you know about her practice?

I have always understood positive thinking is crucial to good health, and that's what I thought this work would be.

What was your opinion of alternative and complementary medicine before working with her?

I had a high regard for it because I believe our Western approach to health uses too many toxins and pharmaceuticals. It seems only to be profit-driven.

What is your opinion of complementary and alternative medicine after doing this work with Dr. Davie?

My opinion has only gotten better. I truly believe thoughts are things. As you think, so you become. (I stole that from Tony Robbins.)

What did you experience while working with her? How did it make you feel?

I experienced a tremendous sense of well-being. It made me feel like I had a chance of beating the cancer.

The most helpful thing about the work I did with Dr. Davie is--

Realizing the importance of forgiveness.

The most difficult part of the work I did with Dr. Davie is--

Truthfully, the most difficult part of working with Dr. Davie was our cell phone connection. Often I could not hear or understand what she was saying, and it made me frustrated. It was no one's fault; it was just a technological problem.

After doing this work, I realized--

The power of the universe and the energy that is present all around.

Doing this work changed the way I--

Look at everything. Whereas in the recent past I preferred to spend my days inside, now I crave the outdoors and see how I'm connected to the universe.

What other non-traditional modalities have you experienced?

Meditation, EMDR, acupuncture, massage, and reflexology.

What other modalities have been helpful to you? Please state how that modality was helpful in your situation.

The honest truth is that I do the other modalities as stated above. How they help me in my condition is unclear, but I have to do them for my peace of mind. And for having stage-4 lung cancer, I feel pretty healthy these days, much better than before I was diagnosed.

In what way or ways have these alternative modalities affected your life?

Now I make time to meditate, and I've slowed down tremendously. My stress levels have decreased in spades.

Do you have any insights or recommendations to people who are considering alternative and holistic modalities?

> I would recommend people try holistic and alternative modalities. It forces you to be 100 percent honest, and you really can't hide, so it cuts to the core of what's real for you.

Do you have any insights or recommendations to share with people who are skeptical about alternative and holistic modalities?

> People generally think this kind of work is voodoo. My plan is to be the person who beats lung cancer holistically, and then help others do the same.

EXERCISE: LOVINGKINDNESS MEDITATION

10-20 minutes

Practicing this lovingkindness meditation has been proven to confer many healthy effects, including migraine relief and increased overall well-being.

Sit in a comfortable position. Bring your attention to your breath. Allow your breath to become slow, long, deep, and comfortable.

Inhale. Pause if you wish. As you breathe out, silently say the following statement:

May I be happy.

Inhale. Pause if you wish. As you breathe out, silently say the following statement:

May I be safe and protected.

Inhale. Pause if you wish. As you breathe out say silently the following statement:

May I be healthy and strong.

Inhale. Pause if you wish. As you breathe out, silently say the following statement:

May I be surrounded with loving friends and family.

Repeat these steps for 2-4 minutes.

Next place your attention on someone you love dearly, and with each breath say silently as you exhale:

May you be happy.

May you be safe and protected.

May you be healthy and strong.

May you be surrounded with loving friends and family.

Repeat these steps for 2-4 minutes.

Next place your attention on a stranger; for example, the clerk at the grocery store or the mailman, and silently repeat for 2-4 minutes as you breathe out:

May you be happy.

May you be safe and protected.

May you be healthy and strong.

May you be surrounded with loving friends and family.

Next place your attention on someone you dislike or have a conflict with and silently repeat 2-4 minutes:

May you be happy.

May you be safe and protected.

May you be healthy and strong.

May you be surrounded with loving friends and family.

Finally, place your attention on a group, such as your whole family, your community, or your town, and repeat for 2-4 minutes:

May we be happy.

May we be safe and protected.

May we be healthy and strong.

May we be surrounded with loving friends and family.

You can continue to place your attention on your whole state, country, and eventually the whole world, repeating these sentences for a few minutes.

Return to watching your breath.

Notice how you feel.

Chapter 14: Janet and Molly

Two Cases of Breast Cancer

I don't get angry; I grow a tumor instead.
— Woody Allen

CASE 1: JANET

Janet, a forty-eight-year-old horse breeder, came to me because of several problems. She recently had surgery for breast cancer, felt anxious, had insomnia, and wrestled with self-esteem issues. In our first session she stated her goals clearly: "I want to be healthier, and I want to be sure the cancer doesn't come back. I want to find some path through the anxiety and sadness I feel."

Beginning with a discussion of her history, I learned about Janet's difficult childhood with a mentally ill mother and a controlling father. In her adult life, however, she loved her work with horses and had built a thriving business. She had been married for eighteen years to a man she loved. But five years earlier she discovered his affair with his childhood sweetheart. She confronted him, and they sought help through therapy. He stopped seeing his ex-girlfriend, apologized for hurting Janet, and re-affirmed his love; yet Janet felt unable to wholly forgive him and move beyond the feelings of betrayal.

Janet asked me to help her feel at peace with herself and her husband. Though she no longer doubted his sincerity and faithfulness, she remained troubled by his affair. Whenever he visited his family—in a city where his ex-girlfriend also lived—Janet stressed out.

Because she wanted to learn how to relax, we worked on her anxiety using breathing exercises and monitoring her heart-rate variability with a **HeartMath** machine (see Glossary). Using energy psychology techniques and Focusing, Janet soon achieved a desirable heart-rate variability. Soon her anxiety resolved and she slept better. She fully forgave her husband and enjoyed a deeper level of intimacy with him. She no longer worried about his travels or past affair.

In addition, we worked on imagery regarding her breast. The darkness Janet initially sensed in her right breast slowly dissolved and transformed into healthy, pink breast tissue. She ate a vegan, live-food diet. She felt energetic and continued to pursue her passion for training and nurturing retired horses.

CASE 2: MOLLY

Molly is a seventy-seven-year-old woman who came to see me with her eighty-one-year-old husband, Bernard, because they both wanted help with several issues. This couple clearly cared about each other. Bernard worried about Molly, who cried easily and unexpectedly; she seemed anxious most of the time, and he wanted her to feel happier. Molly worried about Bernard, who mentally seemed less sharp than he used to be, and she thought he was depressed. He had been working for their son until a few months ago, when he no longer could do the work skillfully, and he was let go. Bernard acknowledged experiencing memory difficulties.

In the first session, both shared their individual medical histories. Neither had seen a doctor or had blood evaluations for several years. They were in between health plans and expected to meet with a new doctor in the next month. They were conscientious about their diet, which included cereals, breads, chicken, vegetables, and fruits. They ate broiled or baked fish, meat, or chicken once a day and did not consume many sweets, fried foods, or alcohol. Neither one smoked. They lived close to family and friends and spent most of their time indoors.

Bernard and Molly took supplements, including a multivitamin, 2000 mg of vitamin D, and fish oils every day. Bernard took a supplement a friend recommended for his memory. He had not noticed a change since he started taking it a month ago. Molly took medications for hypertension and hypothyroidism.

When she told me she was diagnosed with breast cancer twenty years ago, Molly could hardly speak, as if she had a big lump in her throat, and tears ran down her face. Since then, she had felt anxious and cried often, which disturbed Bernard. He tried to console her, giving her back rubs that seemed to be helpful in calming her a little, but her anxiety persisted. He felt like he needed to walk on eggshells, and even then, he didn't know what triggered her distress. He wanted her to feel better but did not know how to comfort her.

I explained that I could help them on several levels: medically, psychologically, and mentally. For medical evaluation, I recommended having blood tests to determine if they had nutritional deficiencies or other medical conditions. I was concerned about vitamin D deficiency and inflammation, which could explain Bernard's memory changes and possibly some depression symptoms. Both conditions are correctable simply with diet and vitamins. I also wanted to know Bernard's ferritin (iron stores) levels. If elevated, that could contribute to inflammation. I taught Molly TFT (Thought Field Therapy, see Glossary), showing her how to use tapping to relieve her anxiety about having had breast cancer. After a few rounds, she spoke more calmly and with fewer tears.

We agreed they would obtain blood test results and then return for another session.

The labs confirmed my suspicion of nutritional deficiencies. Molly and Bernard were deficient in vitamin D; Bernard's ferritin level was slightly elevated, and his blood sugar level indicated he was pre-diabetic—both of which cause inflammation. The couple also registered high levels of homocysteine and C-reactive Protein (CRP), specific indicators of inflammation and possible nutritional deficiency.

I recommended dietary changes, which they felt comfortable with. To address the elevated ferritin, Bernard was to decrease his intake of meat products. They were both to follow an anti-inflammatory diet (see Appendix A) and increase greens and vegetables, lentils, and bean casseroles. I recommended they spend at least fifteen to twenty minutes a day in the sun, as well as take enough vitamin D for one week to restore their reserves, then taking it at a higher maintenance dose for four to six weeks before retesting their vitamin D levels.

Researching the supplement Bernard was taking, which included several ingredients, I discovered the scientific evidence of their efficacy to be conflicting with reports of adverse reactions and possible interference with normal metabolic function. I gave Bernard the scientific information and suggested he consider discontinuing it, based on his experience of lack of benefit and the current research.

In the next session Bernard again accompanied Molly, and he informed me she had been less upset but still cried easily. I suggested Molly have an individual session with me and for Bernard to wait outside.

Molly told me about her childhood, which she described as "good, although we were quite poor." She met Bernard at age nineteen, and a year later they married. They had three children and three grandchildren.

I asked her what had happened the years before she developed breast cancer. Tearing up again, with a lump in her throat, she informed me that Bernard had left her for another woman. However, after her cancer diagnosis, he ended his extramarital relationship and returned to stay with Molly and care for her. He has been with her since, yet after twenty years of being attentive and faithful, she still feared he would leave her.

Using TFT, we worked on her anxiety about having breast cancer, until she felt at peace when she thought about it. She expressed amazement that she could think about her cancer experience and not cry or feel upset; the fear that it might recur had disappeared.

At that point I asked Bernard to join us, and I encouraged Molly to share with Bernard what she told me. For the first time in twenty years, she told him she was afraid he would leave her again. Obviously distressed by her pain, Bernard said he would not leave her. He also explained that, at the time of the affair, he hadn't known what to do, because she had kicked him out of the house and had been mad at him, but that he always loved her. We all tapped about the distress of that time and, with TFT, individually addressed emotions as they came up.

Working through feelings of shame, guilt, anger, and regret, we continued to address each residual emotion and the memories that surfaced. Bernard recalled when he was three, his father left his mother. Bernard had not seen him again until he was a teenager. Even then, he did not feel his father cared enough or loved him; they never truly connected. Bernard had been a well-behaved kid and did his best to avoid stressing his mom, stepfather, and father.

Using TFT, we tapped on Bernard's abandonment by his father, and both he and Molly were surprised he teared up. Molly had never seen Bernard so vulnerable. Now that she saw him cry, she could see a different, softer part of him, and was comforted. Knowing they were safe to access their feelings and share them with love, they were able to communicate their feelings with comfort and ease. When Bernard told Molly, "You're the only one I've ever loved—and I love you now."

Molly apologized for kicking him out. "It was my fault," she said.

"No, it wasn't. You were just going through menopause. I didn't understand that. I didn't know how to help you, so I sort of withdrew."

"I thought you were acting like nothing was happening to me, like you didn't care. I wanted to connect with you on a deeper level, but I gave up on you."

That day they left looking at each other with tenderness and a new, deeper understanding.

In our last session, the couple reported that Bernard's memory was sharper and he was feeling better. Molly's affect was no longer erratic, and she seemed much more relaxed and happy. They felt closer than ever, speaking about feelings and concerns with a better understanding of each other. They planned to follow up with their physician regarding inflammation and vitamin D levels.

A year later, they are happy and are doing well.

DISCUSSION

Cancer is the second leading cause of death for women in the U.S., after heart disease. And in women, lung cancer mortality is two and a half times that of the vastly more prevalent breast cancer. Dr. Hannah Weir of the Centers for Disease Control (CDC) predicts, based upon epidemiological studies, that the incidence of and death rate from lung, breast, and colon cancer will increase over the next few years.

Several factors, most of which have been known for a long time, affect the development of cancer:

- genetics and epigenetics

- diet

- exposure to toxins such as alcohol, pesticides, cigarettes, radiation, and other carcinogens

- and more recently, an elevated ACE score (adverse childhood experiences)

Epigenetics is the science of studying modification of *gene expression* rather than alteration of the genetic code itself. Simply stated, epigenetics investigates the environment surrounding one's genes. The more we learn about this environment and its dynamics, the more health options we find. For example, understanding the interaction between nutrition and epigenetics is critical to identifying breast cancer risk because of the influence of diet during early stages of mammary gland development. Furthermore, a better understanding of epigenetics will lead to better resolution of the common denominators contributing to cancer—childhood traumas, poor nutrition, pesticides, and other substances which promote or induce cancer.

The findings of this relatively new area of research are promising. In my work with cancer patients, I explore the person's entire history, looking for the clues that influence epigenetics—dietary, medical, emotional, and life experiences—and those that will lead to health.

EXERCISE: ANSWERS THROUGH DIVINATION
15-20 minutes

This exercise accesses the subconscious and allows you to look at decision-making in a new light. Try this when you feel conflicted about a choice between two or more actions.

Take a walk in nature while thinking about the issue, and carry a pen and paper with you. Ask a question, such as: Which job should I take? Or should I stick with the job I have?

Observe the stones and rocks as you walk, looking for those that seem particularly interesting. When you see one that calls to you, pick it up.

Look at one side of the rock and write down four descriptive sentences about what you see. For example: I see a pink line; the rock is smooth; I see a triangle; I see the image of a bear.

Next turn the rock over and write four descriptive terms about the other side of the rock.

Then go back to each description you wrote and complete a sentence in writing:

The pink line tells me about this situation that _____.

The triangle tells me about this situation that _____.

The smooth surface tells me about this situation that _____.

The image of the bear tells me that _____.

Do this until you have completed a sentence for all eight descriptions.

Has your understanding of the situation changed?

Chapter 15: Collin

A Case of Suicide

*Let nature be your teacher, let love
be your guide.* – Unattributed

COLLIN SUMMONED TREMENDOUS courage to merely walk
through my door and sit down. Perched on the edge of the
armchair, feet jiggling, he was so nervous he could not utter a
word or look at me. He shook visibly and panted in rapid, shallow breaths. His flushed face and sweaty hands rounded out the
picture of someone in extreme, disabling distress.

Clearly, achieving some level of relaxation was the first priority. I asked him to copy my gestures and repeat after me while
tapping the side of his hand (the "karate chop" point). I recited
for him, "Even though I can't speak and I'm so anxious, I deeply
and completely love and accept myself." On the third repetition of
this affirmation, Collin articulated some words and looked at me,
though without making eye contact. I moved my hands to my face,
tapping on the anxiety acupoint and other relevant acupuncture

points (see the diagram in Appendix B), repeating the sentences with alternate words:

I am so nervous.
I am so anxious.
My hands are sweaty.
I can't speak.
I can't make eye contact.

After a couple of rounds, he told me he felt anxious and suffered panic attacks in social situations. He wanted me to help him be more relaxed. I asked him when the panic attacks had begun and how he usually coped with them in his life. He replied that for years he simply had used avoidance and self-isolation to deal with these episodes.

Using hypnosis, I guided him to imagine a safe place. First he chose a golf course at dusk, but he switched to a dog park with grass, where he felt a soft breeze, heard the rustling leaves, and smelled fresh pines in the cool, crisp air, still wet from rain. There he felt relaxed and safe, and he manifested that feeling in my office.

After several minutes in this trance, I asked him to notice what in his life prevented him from feeling safe and relaxed. Collin described tension in his torso and a sensation of being stuck. He shared a concern about being inadequate in his marriage. "My wife is beautiful, confident, and successful. We met ten years ago in college, when we were young and idealistic. She took my breath away, but I felt she was too beautiful to ever be interested in me."

Nonetheless, they became friends. She made the first move toward a more intimate relationship. Over the years, she matured and became a skilled professional, and Collin supported her growth. But as she became more confident and self-sufficient, he felt that he continued to flounder. "I don't know who I am," he said. He expressed profound shame and guilt.

I learned Collin had graduated from college and worked as a writer. Because of a lack of work, though, he began attending business school, where he felt like the oddball in the class. He thought and behaved differently. He didn't speak up. A fellow student's jibes humiliated him.

After setting an intention and prayer for healing for the highest good, with safety and ease, I guided him into a light trance and asked him to focus on life, living, and loving himself.

He took a deep breath but still looked troubled. "I don't want to live," he said, adding calmly, "My father gave me a gun some time ago, and I plan to use it to kill myself."

In the face of this unexpected declaration, I remained present and accepting of all of him. I employed the Subjective Units of Discomfort Scale (SUDS) to measure the intensity of his feelings. I asked him to rate his agreement with the following statements on a scale of zero to ten—ten being completely true and zero being not true at all:

"I want to live." Response: 2/10.

"I want to die." Response: 8/10.

"I accept love." Response: 5/10.

"I accept healing." Response: 5/10.

He expressed his intentions and feelings calmly, still in the trance. With only fifteen minutes left to the session, this finding changed the situation; time no longer was a limiting factor. I understood that Collin, beyond being depressed, was dangerously suicidal (80 percent), had little will to live (20 percent), and felt despair, as he was not wholly accepting love and healing (50 percent). He admitted thinking about suicide for a few weeks.

Again I invited him to notice the feeling elicited in his body as I made certain statements. He experienced discomfort in his chest, as if trapped, constricted, and in pain.

A memory surfaced: "I awoke in a foul mood, tried to write,

and I couldn't," Collin recalled. "I felt like an injured animal and couldn't escape the suffering. I felt disconnected from myself."

Continuing our process, his breathing relaxed more. He forgave some people who had hurt him, including some he was surprised to remember.

We continued for another hour until he felt free of the negative feelings contributing to his wish to die. When I felt we had reached a safe and stable place, I asked him what he chose to replace his panic and negative feelings with. He chose what he wanted for himself at that moment: to live and be with his wife.

We re-tested, using SUDS, with vastly different results:

"I want to live." Response: 10/10
"I want to die." Response: 0/10.
"I accept love." Response: 10/10.
"I accept healing." 10/10.

It is important to note the SUDS scale, which relies on the client's own assessments, is subjective; yet it is nonetheless reliable in showing emotional change because of the before-and-after evaluations. Clearly, Collin's feelings had shifted significantly. I next proceeded to help him integrate and mark that place of well-being so he could access it on his own.

Collin looked like a new person. He stood taller and reported, "I feel I have my life back." After making an appointment for the following week, he promised in a contract with me that he would seek help if needed and would not harm himself.

A week later, he reported no suicidal thoughts. He had disposed of the gun. We worked together regularly for two months, and Collin increasingly felt much better. He learned to use EFT to release his anxiety. He had discontinued taking antidepressants months before our sessions (because of the expense and the way it made him feel); without them, he felt as if a cloud had been lifted. He could feel the emotions that had been numbed. He felt more alive.

However, he remained afraid to be depressed and have an unhappy life, like his father. So even though he no longer felt suicidal, he experienced symptoms of depression. We worked on both his depression and other issues of low self-esteem, anxiety, shame, and guilt. Many of those resolved and were replaced with confidence, trust, self-esteem, and satisfaction. At home, his wife noticed his new self-confidence.

Collin's feeling of depression entirely resolved after working on a few childhood memories, including a time he almost drowned and felt shame and fear as a result of his father's reaction when he saved him. I cannot say what the relevance of this memory was, just that it triggered a significant shift in Collin's expression and brought a smile and a look of relief to his face. He expressed an awareness that the depression belonged to his father, and he did not have to own it. He could let it go and be free to be his own person. Five years later, Collin remains free of depression and is doing well.

Discussion

Dealing with an acutely suicidal person who was suffering and in despair, right in my office, marked a first for me. If I had just relied upon my medical school training and conventional knowledge, I would not have trusted the process I used. Instead, as an emergency physician, I would have consulted with psychiatry to evaluate and treat him. He likely would have been admitted and medicated, and it would be unlikely for him to achieve the transformation he actually experienced.

This is a key distinction in the work I do today in integrative psychology versus the medicine I practiced as an emergency physician: the paradigm has changed, and spontaneous healing is possible. While Collin's depression had been evaluated and his *symptoms* were treated over the course of his college years, his health and well-being had worsened to the point of feeling suicidal.

That day of his first visit, my inner guidance told me I could treat his emotional state the same way I would treat any other problem. Looking back, not for one minute did I question my intervention. During the session, I felt the trust Collin placed in me as well as the trust I had in the process and in Collin as a human being capable of healing. All felt transparent and clear, without fear or doubt.

When I work with individuals, I am in a deep, focused state of awareness where I use all my senses. I become in tune with the client, and together we embark on an emotional, spiritual, and physical journey—akin to what runners often feel: one with the earth, one with the wind, at peace. I enter a harmonious state that allows me to be in the present moment, and that moment feels expansive and inclusive. Compare this path toward healing to the more common method of treating symptoms. Taking an aspirin or other pain medication decreases the inflammatory substances causing a pain sensation or stimulating pain neurons. But pain medications do not fix the origin of the pain and its root cause. Unless these are resolved, complete healing does not occur.

With ill health, the body and mind are out of balance, so treating the symptoms is often inadequate. Full health is a more likely outcome when you summon the natural power of the body and mind to heal and re-balance. When this is achieved, any medical prognosis becomes irrelevant, because health and balance are restored.

The techniques I used did not heal Collin. Those modalities no doubt were strategic in facilitating the healing, but ultimately Collin's inner knowing and innate resources brought healthful balance back to his mind and body. I cannot over-emphasize the importance of our individual power to heal.

Also of note is that Collin came with severe anxiety; when the troubling emotion subsided sufficiently, the suicidal intention that surfaced was more pressing and more important to address than his initial symptom. This is a common phenomenon (also known as the *tooth-shoe-lump* principle.) Often when someone has a strong emotion, other emotions may also be present, but they may not come forward until the overpowering emotion decreases. That is why people may feel worse when working with a therapist on an issue. The uppermost problem may only be a small part of a greater, more serious issue, or it may mask another. When this happens, a skilled therapist has the opportunity to help resolve whatever surfaces and to turn obstacles into steppingstones.

Exercise: Being present,
using the fronto-occipital hold
5-10 minutes

Think of a situation that concerns you or may be causing some distress. Notice how you feel about it, with acceptance and without judgment.

Where do you feel it in your body?

What is its shape, color, and feel?

Does it have a sound or carry a message?

How does "it" feel—sad, angry, tired? Acknowledge whatever comes to your awareness.

Take a slow, deep breath.

Go into the fronto-occipital hold for 3-10 minutes (see the diagram in Appendix B), putting your attention on whatever comes up and accepting that.

Notice how you feel about this situation now. Has anything changed? How does it feel in your body?

Chapter 16: Christopher

A Case of PTSD

The distinction between past, present,
and future is only an illusion, even if
a stubborn one. – Albert Einstein

FOR EACH OF US, the steppingstones of our history pave our path forward. Often this appears to be linear, but sometimes very little separates the past and the present, especially in regard to trauma. Though current circumstances are widely different from the childhood onset of trauma, both may be experienced exactly the same way.

Christopher, a forty-four-year-old professional, called me and asked for help with a prolonged, extreme case of panic. His voice shook as he spoke, and I reassured him I could help if he would commit to several months of work to permanently resolve his post-traumatic stress disorder (PTSD). He agreed, and we scheduled a long initial session to clear his panicked state.

On September 16, 2014, wearing shorts and a T-shirt, Christopher staggered into my office and collapsed into the armchair, stuttering: "I'm a wreck!" His sweat-stained face was as red as a radish, his T-shirt was soaked, he looked haggard, and his eyes flared wide, like a terrified animal's.

Needing to calm him before taking a history, I started by asking him to copy me. Tapping on the side of the hand, I said, "Even though I am terribly anxious, I deeply and completely love and accept myself."

Christopher stuttered as he said it, shaking as he tapped on the karate chop point.

I continued: "Even though I am terribly anxious and I can't talk or walk straight, I deeply and completely love and accept myself."

Christopher echoed my words and copied my actions as I proceeded with various acupoints. I used different phrases to address many of his symptoms:

Even though I'm distressed, I deeply and completely love and accept myself.

. . . trembling . . .

. . . staggering . . .

. . . can't speak . . .

. . . can't walk . . .

. . . can't sleep . . .

. . . can't work . . .

. . . so anxious . . .

When his breathing slowed a bit and his shaking was less intense, Christopher was able to blurt out some of the history pertaining to this panic attack. Since 2001, when the World Trade Center buildings collapsed, Christopher experienced this panic for a week around each 9/11 anniversary. He said the current episode was the worst ever, and he despaired of ever being free of them.

I also learned that for a week he had been taking Xanax, commonly prescribed for anxiety, and he typically drank four to five glasses of wine in the evening. Also, his girlfriend had difficulty dealing with Christopher's situation.

His thoughts raced as he blurted out more information:

My world is up in the air.

My mother left when I moved close to her.

She's bipolar.

I need to move away.

My heart, it's racing.

My chest hurts.

I directed him to put his attention on what he felt in his chest while I asked several questions:

"What does the feeling in your chest look like?" *A cloud of burning lava.*

"If it could make a sound, what would you hear?" *High-pitched squeal.*

"What would it taste like?" *Chalk.*

"What would it smell like?" *Chalk.*

"What would it feel like?" *Frenetic.*

I guided him into a light trance. He continued shaking. I spoke softly: "You don't have to do anything except put your attention on what I am going to say. You can rest with your eyes closed."

I guided him through the intention for the work, including a prayer, affirming the healing would be for his highest good, and it would happen with ease and grace, with the protection of a higher source, and it would be complete. He took a breath.

As I continued, he took a longer breath, like a sigh, and relaxed even more. When I asked him how he felt, he said, "It's better."

We resumed the process, more comfortably, and I continued to hold the space for his healing, articulating what he had already expressed.

Slowly, his shoulders relaxed a bit as he sighed again.

He reported feeling relieved. "The cloud is dispersing," he said. "Just a little burning remains."

Christopher began sharing more information. He said pensively, with a trace of a smile: "Chewing tobacco." I repeated that, and he smiled. I understood chewing tobacco comforted him, and he was beginning to feel that comfort. I did not need to know more, only enough to help him continue. We were going in the right direction.

He now looked a lot more relaxed and said his chest didn't feel so tight. He expressed wanting to spend more quality time with family. He drank some water, describing a feeling like a cool breeze. He wiped sweat from his forehead.

The time had come to free Christopher from the pain, the hurt, resentment, and being stuck. I explained forgiveness does not mean *condoning* anything, it just means *accepting* what has happened and that it's over. Then I told him a story about forgiveness.

He relaxed further, as tears streamed down his face. He said, "Snot tastes better when you cry," and laughed. "I feel another cool breeze. I haven't felt nice like this for a week. Thank you."

He swallowed several big gulps of water, and sighed. He yawned. After two hours of deep work, Christopher looked perfectly relaxed, and I knew he needed to rest.

I asked him to choose something positive and meaningful to carry with him in his thoughts and his heart.

"I choose forgiveness."

With a smile on his face and his hands resting on his heart, no longer sweating, I helped him integrate the deep work. His eyes were bright, and he shook my hand in gratitude as we scheduled the next appointment in two weeks.

During the next session, I obtained more history. He told me his understanding of the trauma underlying his panic attack. He worked at the World Trade Center in 2001. Six days before the 9/11 attacks, he was transferred to California. Very early on the morning of the 11th, while he talked on the phone to a colleague at the World Trade Center, the communication suddenly stopped. Soon thereafter, he heard about planes crashing into the towers. Severely distressed, Christopher left work and headed home. After some time he learned all sixty-seven of his coworkers in NY had perished. Not one survived. Worse, one of his subordinates, a father with several children, had asked Christopher to approve a business trip outside NY, but he had refused. Had Christopher approved the trip, the man would not have died, and Christopher felt doubly guilty for his responsibility in this man's death.

We began by focusing on the guilt he carried for surviving his sixty-seven colleagues and specifically for the subordinate who had requested to travel. We worked to clear his guilt, anger, distress, and sadness about the tragedy. By the end of the session, he forgave himself and accepted forgiveness.

During our next session, I informed him that for him to have had such a severe reaction to 9/11, thirteen years after it happened, meant he had childhood traumas he needed to heal. I asked him to talk about his childhood and to list all the traumas he could remember. There were several.

- His older stepbrother and sister repeatedly attacked and beat him.

- His bipolar mother chased him with a knife.

- His strict father belted him.

- Alcohol dependence was prevalent among family members.

- His parents fought and divorced when he was young.

- He had several motor vehicle accidents as a teenager.

Christopher had worked with a psychotherapist for eleven years, who attributed his problems to his parents, chiefly his father. His father lived in another state and "knew how to push" Christopher's buttons. Whenever they met for holidays or other occasions, they would fight. It only took a couple of hours before Christopher would feel angry and alienated. I listened compassionately.

I asked Christopher about his nutrition and substance use. He regularly drank four to six glasses of wine at night and chewed tobacco. In his youth he used to do cocaine but had stopped a long time ago.

Among his enjoyments, he listed having sex with his girlfriend, running, hiking, and being in nature with his dogs. He loved his girlfriend, but they often fought. She would "provoke" him and "threaten to call the police," which she had done. The police actually arrested him once.

Appreciating his courage to share his history, I invited him to relax in the armchair, take a deep breath, and let go of everything that had happened in the past few minutes. I guided him to feel the relaxation in each part of his body as we progressed through releasing everything from the past hour, the past day, the past week, the past month, the past year—all the way to letting go of everything that had happened. I guided him to a place of safety and peace, near a lake in nature, among pine trees, with his dog.

From this place, we began addressing the issues interfering with his state of peace and comfort, one at a time. When the two hours were over, Christopher had shed tears and felt relief and forgiveness for himself and others.

Over the next couple of months, we addressed his triggers, anger, and relationship issues with his father. He realized how much he loved his father and wanted to get closer to him. That Thanksgiving, Christopher visited his family. He reported that some of the past provocations now tended to amuse him. He did not get as angry at many of his dad's comments that would have previously led to a verbal fight. He experienced them for what they were: comments he disagreed with rather than triggers. He no longer felt like he had to win the argument with his father.

Though not free of anger, he felt he was learning to recognize its onset and look at the situation differently or leave the scene before his anger got out of control. He realized he had to give himself a chance to recognize and accept his emotions so they wouldn't hijack him to a place he did not wish to go. He felt empowered and proud of himself.

For the next four months, Christopher remained free of panic attacks. He enjoyed a pattern of feeling quiet and relaxed, in particular after our sessions, and a solid night's sleep followed. It is not unusual for a person to feel tired after doing deep work in a session that clears earlier trauma, even though he or she may have been unaware of their deeper emotions.

Nevertheless, one afternoon Christopher called to ask for help in between our sessions. He had not slept for three nights; the panic attack was persistent and relentless; his breath was shallow and rapid, his heart raced, and his palms felt cold and sweaty; he felt unsteady on his feet and could not walk straight; his speech reflected his highly anxious state—just as he had presented when he first came to see me.

Over the telephone, I guided him through breathing exercises for about twelve minutes, until he felt a little better. The pitch of his voice returned to normal, and he spoke without hesitation or self-correction. He took more air into his lungs and his breathing slowed more. We set the intention with a prayer for our session: to do the healing work for Christopher's highest good, especially the parts of him feeling anxious, scared, and conflicted, and that the healing happen safely, with ease and grace.

Christopher described the evening his panic attack began. His girlfriend had just left town to visit her family, and he sat down in his recliner after dinner to watch a game of golf on TV. He couldn't say why, but he began to feel anxious and could not sleep that night or the following two nights. He found he couldn't run in the daytime, an activity that usually helped him sleep well. The morning of his call, he was feeling the full-blown symptoms of a panic attack for the first time in several months. He could not abort the attack on his own.

I listened to the description of his symptoms—his fear and angst, the tightness in his chest—and I guided him to connect to a memory of these same feelings in his childhood. He remembered a time when he was six years old and his home felt like "cowboys and Indians." His mom and dad were fighting, and the house "felt like a war zone."

We started clearing the emotional scar of this traumatic memory. Christopher initially relaxed a little, but then his fear and anxiety spiked higher. Now he remembered a time when he was three or four years old and feared going to sleep because, "If I went to sleep, I would not be able to breathe." He felt this fear in his "bones." Exploring this further, he related stories of abuse by his older stepsiblings.

Integrating various energy psychology techniques, I helped him clear the scars of trauma. He felt better almost immediately. Christopher laughed and said, "I feel eighteen million times better!" That night he slept soundly.

As we continued the work—a total of twenty hours over six months—Christopher connected on a deep level with his father. He spent several weeks with him, caring for him during a heath crisis. He stopped drinking alcohol. Christopher acknowledged being content, and he made plans to move to another state.

Almost two years later, Christopher faced another challenge

and resumed self-medicating with alcohol. His stepbrother, diagnosed with amyotrophic lateral sclerosis (ALS, also known as Lou Gehrig's disease), deteriorated rapidly over the course of a few months, going from hiking in the mountains to being wheelchairbound. Christopher supported his stepbrother and spent much time with him. However, his stepbrother was severely depressed and drank heavily. Christopher returned to drinking in response to this situation, but he soon realized he no longer liked the effects of alcohol, he could be in charge of his life, and drinking did not support his stepbrother. He again chose to stop drinking, joined Alcoholics Anonymous, and took time off to take care of himself by spending a great deal of time in nature and joining a meditation group.

Christopher now is doing very well, feeling like a whole new person. He meditates and does yoga regularly within his busy professional schedule.

Discussion

Post-traumatic stress disorder, commonly known as PTSD, has been recognized to result from experiencing or witnessing severe, often life-threatening trauma. In the U.S., there are eight million documented cases of PTSD; I suspect the actual number is much higher. People with PTSD may not seek help or medical attention because they may be afraid of the stigma of mental and psychological disorders. Furthermore, when in a state of shock or hypervigilance, they are less likely to seek help or trust that someone can help them.

Affected individuals experience hyper-vigilance, anxiety, panic, depression, insomnia, recurrent nightmares, flashbacks, terror, and may self-medicate with drugs and alcohol. They often display behavior that is considered aggressive and antisocial. They typically wrestle with shame, guilt, and anger. It is not unusual to dissociate the memory of the event and the symptoms. In the case of Christopher, he developed PTSD after 9/11, and his symptoms worsened with the years.

Individuals with adverse childhood experiences (ACE) are more likely to develop PTSD after a traumatic event. Christopher had at least four categories of adverse childhood experiences: physical abuse, a family member with a mental health problem, alcohol use by a family member, and parental divorce. This predisposed him to developing PTSD.

Self-medicating with alcohol and drugs relieved many symptoms but did not clear the problem. Moreover, Christopher had eleven years of therapy with continued and increasing symptoms of PTSD. Conventional therapy did not cure his PTSD. Medication with pharmaceuticals (such as Xanax) also may numb the symptoms, but unless the scars of the original traumas are addressed effectively, the problem persists and continues to worsen. Only when the specific traumas were addressed on several levels did Christopher begin to heal.

Why did a panic attack happen while watching a game of golf on TV? Was it related to his girlfriend leaving for a couple of days? What triggered it? In my opinion, the coexistence of several occurrences sparked a subconscious response to a childhood memory that had scarred him. Most likely the immediate stimulus was a scene on TV, possibly a commercial, maybe a word or tone of voice. But Christopher also suffered from severe PTSD and erratic sleep. So, though his awareness was in the present, his subconscious mind responded as if he were experiencing the childhood trauma when he was six, and then earlier when he was three. To young Christopher, it was much better to stay awake in fear than to sleep and risk suffocation and death. As his subconscious took charge of his actions and feelings—all without him consciously remembering those incidents—there suddenly was no difference between his present and his past. He only knew his body and mind felt hijacked.

Through our work he realized his fear and anxiety had protected him from falling asleep and being vulnerable to further abuse. This protective reaction helped him survive, and it remained stored in his subconscious, ready to be activated in perceived threatening situations. Christopher became able to heal from trauma when he recalled to consciousness the earlier traumatic memory: he realized he was a grown man; he no longer feared his stepbrother, who would no longer harm him; and his reaction no longer served him in the present.

Similarly, he consciously knew 9/11 existed in the past and no longer presented a danger, yet he experienced severe panic attacks with palpitations, shaking, inability to care for himself, sweating, and insomnia. When we addressed and uncoupled the past event from his current situation, the underlying issues of shock, shame, and guilt emerged, making it possible for Christopher to free himself of them.

Dealing with a panic attack without treating the underlying traumas does not resolve the problem—in fact, it may exacerbate it. It's like putting a band-aid on an infected wound, because there is a splinter under the skin—the band-aid helps neither the wound nor the infection. Only removing the splinter will facilitate healing. Even taking aspirin or antibiotics won't help. They abate the symptoms but do not address the true problem.

Christopher healed by moving into a place of acceptance, love, and forgiveness. He could relax. That night, he slept peacefully, recognizing he was safe and no longer vulnerable.

A few years later, Christopher continues to do well and feels at peace, filled with love and optimism. He informs me another benefit he experienced from our work together is that for the past few years, he has not experienced a bout of ulcerative colitis or needed any medication for this condition, which had troubled him for years. He feels wholly cured.

EXERCISE: ASK AND RECEIVE
WITH FELT SENSE FOR FORGIVENESS
5-15 minutes

Think of someone you would like to forgive but have not been able to do so.

Say: *I forgive [use their name].*

Notice the sensation that comes up. Is it telling you that you have not forgiven? Where in your body do you feel this? What does it feel like? What do you feel? Say the following out loud slowly:

There is a part of my being that already knows how to heal and release this feeling in my [chest, neck, etc.], all its roots, its point of entry, and what it represents from my body, mind, and personal space.

This part of my being is willing to inform the rest of me now.

It is doing so with grace and ease.

My mind, body, and spirit are receiving this information now.

Information transfer is now complete.

Notice what happens now when you repeat: *I forgive [name].*

Notice what you feel. Has the sensation changed? Have you forgiven a little? Not at all? Completely? Your body will let you know. If you feel discomfort, perhaps in a new area, put your attention on it and repeat the statements above. Hopefully you will feel a shift or be able to forgive.

Notice how you feel now when you think about the person or situation.

Chapter 17: Marilyn

A Case of Depression

Every single day say yes to life
(and don't be afraid to say no in
order to do that). – Brian Andreas

L IKE PANIC ATTACKS, depression can be tenacious and complex. Marilyn sought my help to deal with her depression, which she could not free herself of, even with antidepressants. She could not remember a time when she wasn't depressed, and as a child she cried a lot. Now, at age sixty-four, depression overwhelmed her life and relationships.

Marilyn grew up in a poor, devout Catholic family. As the second of nine children, she helped raise her brothers and sisters. She attended Catholic school, where the nuns were strict and unkind. Once a nun falsely accused her of stealing, which caused her to feel powerless and betrayed. She did not feel a connection to the patriarchal God she was supposed to revere.

At age nineteen, she married a man twice her age who had four children. She raised them and her own son, born in their first year of marriage. Her husband was an alcoholic, and the relationship lasted nine years. She waited until his children were grown before deciding to leave him. She also adopted an eighteen-year-old.

Marilyn believed she needed to care for everyone and was responsible for their happiness. She felt guilt for being depressed and unable to feel better. "The price one pays for being alive is to suffer," she said; she did not deserve to live if she did not suffer.

In the first session I guided her to a place of comfort and peace next to the ocean, where she sat on a wicker chair with beautiful, colorful cushions. A few happy clouds floated in a blue sky. The soft sand sparkled in the sun. She felt moisture in the cool breeze. She could hear the birds sing and enjoyed the rhythmic sound of the ocean. She smelled roses, lilacs, and salt in the air. Her chest opened and moved with the ocean. She felt peaceful and free of sadness.

"What in your life prevents you from feeling this peaceful feeling inside?" I asked.

"Guilt," she replied. "I don't do enough. I can't come out of depression and do what I need to do for others. I've been taking antidepressants for twenty-five years, but I continue to feel worse."

We explored her thoughts and beliefs and how they affected her physically. She experienced them in her body as physical sensations of chest tightness and soreness in her throat. Tears ran down her face as she connected with painful emotions. Her sense of guilt intensified, accompanied by a critical voice saying that she never did enough.

She talked about her son, a crack addict. She had kicked him out of the house when he was a teenager and felt severe guilt about having done so. Now he lived in a tent on her property, and she felt more depressed, guilty, and powerless to help him. She loved him dearly and wanted the best for him. It pained her to watch him be self-destructive. She wanted to help him and struggled with her emotions.

I guided her through energy psychology processes while she put her attention on the bodily sensations of the feelings of guilt and depression. Marilyn reported a lessening of the tension, self-reproach, and sadness, and she felt an increasing sense of expansion. She realized she had been a good mother, she did the best she could, and her son's addiction was not her fault. At the end of the session she felt love and peace. "I feel God," she said, marveling. "I haven't had that feeling for a long time."

In the following session, she reported feeling less sadness over the week. Her son was going through a crisis, but she had felt more empowered, able to be present with him without taking responsibility for his problems.

Still, I sensed something oppressive in her mood. "What do you feel in this moment?" I asked.

She replied, "Overwhelming sadness."

Exploring this further, she described being in a dark, foggy, and bitter place. Her chest felt heavy and blocked. "I hold this heaviness like a baby, a two-month-old crying baby who buries its face in my chest."

I encouraged her to hold this baby close to her heart and rock it. Marilyn said it quieted and fell asleep. Her chest relaxed a little and her throat felt some ease and comfort.

Marilyn realized *she* needed comfort and acceptance. At the same time, she was aware that throughout her life she provided comfort and acceptance to everyone else: her first husband and his children, her family, her brothers and sisters. She saw herself taking care of little babies, children, and grown children, holding them with love, caring for them, and nurturing them. She even took care of her mother the way she took care of her baby brothers and sisters. Her mother had been sensitive and fragile, and she took it upon herself to care for her.

As we continued our work, Marilyn no longer felt she needed

to hold babies and comfort them. She felt fulfilled and freed. The tightness and heaviness in her chest dissolved. Her heart was opening.

After six weeks, love and gratitude filled her instead of sadness, and she no longer believed she needed to suffer. Not only did she recognize that she no longer needed to take care of babies, her mother, or her brothers and sisters—she understood *they did not need her to sacrifice herself for them.*

At the two-month mark, Marilyn said, "I'm not stuck in a dark place any more." She felt more mobile. Yet she now carried a compelling fear that her husband might die. They had been married forty years, and she loved him dearly. This fear overwhelmed her. What would become of her? How would she live? How could she tolerate life if he passed away? She kept thinking of him not being there for her. She was afraid that when he passed away she would never get out of bed, that she could not keep on living.

I asked about her husband's health and learned he had no medical problems. No rational basis to her worries existed; she couldn't explain them. "My mind takes off on thoughts about death and blots out everything else."

"When in your life have you experienced this before?" I asked. She remembered being four years old, worrying about her mother falling on the train tracks and dying. She thought of her parents, her siblings who were ill and not doing well, and she thought of herself getting older and dying. Hopelessness engulfed her. Death made life seem meaningless—*why bother?*

After listening attentively, I asked her to again go into her body and notice how these feelings manifested. She again felt heaviness in her chest and darkness. She mentioned her strict Catholic upbringing and feeling sinful. "I'm a bad person and deserve to suffer in order to exist. Living means suffering and lack of suffering means death."

Far from being discouraged at the recurrence of her deep-seated belief, I felt optimism that we would work on this troubling, lifelong feeling. I guided her through tapping on acupoints while stating her beliefs until she could accept herself. Though her hopelessness eased during the session, Marilyn continued over the weeks to feel she deserved to suffer.

We continued to work for about three months, focusing on the many facets of her suffering. Every time she cleared a negative belief, something else came up that demanded attention and became another hurdle to overcome. Overall, however, she felt her condition was improving, and she enjoyed more moments of beauty, gratitude, and freedom while in nature.

She learned to use TFT to self-treat and release negative emotions. Slowly, she let go of many of her negative beliefs, which allowed her to maintain positive thoughts. She could consistently feel good enough, deserving of life without strife, and maintain her feelings of acceptance and happiness.

A couple of months after our work concluded, she decided to take care of a baby. She told me he brought her much joy, energy, and happiness. Four years later, she remains happy. She is healthy and continues to use TFT to help herself and feel gratitude for this boy who came into her life. She lives with her husband, who is also in good health.

DISCUSSION

Depression may be caused by a multitude of factors, and it can take many forms and manifest in various ways. In Marilyn's case, there were traumas, guilt, self-blame, self-doubt, and negative beliefs that may have helped her survive as a child with hardships, but they did not serve her as an adult.

Marilyn engaged with others as a caretaker and nurturer all her life. She sacrificed and suffered, carrying other people's burdens and worrying about them. Although during her therapy she felt better and made some progress, deeper issues surfaced. Just like peeling an onion, layer after layer needed to be addressed, until resolved.

It is interesting that, once she cleared her depression and negative thoughts, she took in another child and found joy and fulfillment—caretaking was basic to her nature, and now she could enjoy doing it without suffering.

Depression is a serious condition, and its impact is not only emotional. It has been associated with heart disease, heart attacks, and other health problems. I was not surprised that Marilyn frequently located her disturbed feelings in her heart. Depression and heart disease have also been associated with adverse childhood experiences (ACE). In my opinion, releasing the depression and the pain and suffering of negative beliefs is likely to lessen the risk of heart disease. Studies have shown that stress increases the risk of heart disease and heart attacks; it is also common medical teaching.

Using antidepressants (SSRIs) also is associated with a higher risk of death from sudden cardiac arrest (see the Wayne Ray article, listed in Appendix D). In my opinion, this can be attributed to the association of depression with a state of inflammation. Furthermore, using antidepressants changes the hormonal milieu and one's general mood, but it does not change the root cause of the depression or the inflammatory state. In fact, using antidepressants or anxiolytics during trauma is associated with a higher incidence of PTSD. In his book, *The Body Keeps the Score*, Bessel van der Kolk reports how traumatic life experiences can manifest as physical and mental problems, which do not resolve until the imprint of the original trauma is resolved.

For many, it is much easier to take a pill and live with limited, and limiting, results. But those dedicated to the restoration of full health show up for inner work, allow themselves to be vulnerable, and accept—and expect—that the work can be life changing.

EXERCISE: RAINBOW MEDITATION
10-18 minutes

This meditation is common to many indigenous cultures, including Native American, Hindu (chakra meditation), and Asian (Qi Gong).

Sit comfortably or lie down on your back with your arms a few inches away from the body, palms up, and feet spread shoulder-width apart. (This can also be done as a standing meditation.)

Notice your breathing.

Imagine a warm, red cloud of light next to you.

With the next inhale, imagine breathing in the warm, red light of the cloud and infusing your whole body with its warmth and color. Enjoy this for two to three breaths, until your whole body is filled with this warm, red energy/light.

With the next exhale, release all the red color until it has cleared from your body. Take a natural breath.

Next imagine an orange cloud of light next to you. Repeat the steps above with this orange cloud. When you have exhaled and it is gone from your body, take a natural breath.

Apply the same process to a cloud of yellow, with the brightness of the sun.

And then imagine a spring-green cloud next to you.

Now imagine a turquoise cloud next to you, enjoying the turquoise color for a couple of breaths. Take a natural breath when you have exhaled the turquoise from your body.

Imagine a purple cloud of light next to you, and repeat the steps of inhaling and exhaling. Take a natural breath.

Finally, imagine a cloud of white light next to you, or any color you desire. Inhale it in your body. Fill your body with this light. *Keep this light within you.*

Chapter 18: Elena and Amy

A Case of End-of-life Issues

Clinical decisions should be based on the
patient's values, not mine (the physician)
. . . . I should never assume the patient
shares my values. — H. Brownell Wheeler, MD

ELENA, A CHAPLAIN and community spiritual healer, contacted me for help regarding Amy, a widow in her late eighties. The two had been friends for over thirty years, and when Amy was diagnosed with Alzheimer's disease two years prior, Elena also became Amy's ombudsman.

In the year before they came to see me, Amy's independence significantly eroded. She could no longer drive, prepare meals, take medications as directed, or be alone for extended periods of time. She needed 24/7 care and was no longer safe living alone. An aide, who came every day for four to six hours, assisted Amy with some of her daily tasks, and Elena consistently accompanied Amy to doctor's appointments, comforted her, and helped manage her everyday needs.

Amy had reached the point at which she was entirely dependent on others—a point at which she previously had determined to end her life. At the outset of her Alzheimer's diagnosis, Amy decided she did not want to live if she were incapable of caring for herself; nor did she want to live in an institution. She would end her life before she reached that stage, and Elena had agreed to help and support her in carrying out this resolution. Amy planned to stop eating and drinking to end her life, and Elena felt comfortable helping her as long as Amy remained aware and able to make decisions.

Now, with Amy's deteriorating independence, there seemed to be only two options: to move into an institutional living arrangement or to consciously end her life. But Amy was not making a decision. When asked if she wanted to end her life, she answered that she *did* want to end her life but did not yet feel *ready*. This left Elena in a bind as to what to do to help her friend, and she feared the time soon would arrive when Amy could no longer give her valid consent to be helped to die.

When Elena contacted me and explained her plight, I could see how it pained her. I felt compassion for this devoted friend who wanted to help honor Amy's wishes, but she also listened to her own moral and spiritual values. I explained that although I practiced energy psychology, I wanted to make sure there were no medical solutions to the problem I needed to consider.

Elena showed me Amy's lab reports and medications. She took thyroid hormones for hypothyroidism, cardiac medications for her heart, important supplements and multi-vitamins, including methylcobalamin, and other drugs for various conditions and symptoms. She followed a wholesome diet Elena prepared for her, which included fresh vegetables and fruits, vitamins, and healthy fats. Several recent medical, neurological, and psychological workups showed Amy had been medically evaluated for treatable causes of dementia. I felt satisfied her medical issues had been addressed.

When Amy and Elena arrived for their session, I met a well-groomed, well-cared for woman, but her facial expression was blank. She also exhibited slow choreiform movements—involuntary motions of her hands and fingers. Frequently she also moved her tongue outside her mouth and smacked her lips. She did not seem aware of these behaviors, but she did indicate her awareness of her situation and verbalized the following:

- I know I am deteriorating mentally and physically.
- I do not wish to live life knowing I might not be aware of my surroundings or be able to understand my situation.
- I want to end my life.
- I do not feel ready to end my life yet.
- I do not know what I need.

Listening carefully and appreciating Amy's and Elena's dilemmas, I explained my job was not to influence Amy to make a decision but rather to allow her to access inner wisdom and guidance and to be at peace.

I asked Amy, "Do you want me to help you figure out what you need?"

She did, and so we set the intention for the work we were about to do. Elena helped Amy into a comfortable seated position, and I spoke out loud the prayer and intention to do healing work for Amy's highest good, with God's help and protection.

I focused my attention on helping Amy be at peace with life and with death. We worked on her acceptance of herself and loving herself, using a combination of modalities. At the end of the session, Amy appeared less agitated and a little more relaxed. We scheduled her return in a week.

In the second session, Elena reported the first session helped calm Amy, but that effect disappeared after two days, when her agitation and anxiety returned. They had visited a few local residential facilities, and none of them satisfied Amy. Afterward, both women felt depressed.

Amy repeated that she wanted to end her life but was not ready to enact her choice. I again started with setting an intention and prayer for healing, stating we were doing the work for her highest good, which included all her family, her loved ones, especially her children, and those involved in her life or situation. Amy had three grown children who lived outside the state.

Gently, I again asked her what troubled her. She didn't know, but she felt it in her chest, in her heart, and in her throat. We worked on these feelings, messages of inner wisdom rising to her awareness, and what needed to heal to bring peace. Elena sat close to her, encouraging her and helping her to feel more comfortable and relaxed.

I began yawning, which told me we were moving deeper toward the source of her troubles. (My yawns indicate the energy is shifting and that the client is processing important issues.)

When I mentioned forgiveness, Amy stayed silent for a time. I waited, and she said, "I need to ask forgiveness from Jody, my daughter."

"Do you feel comfortable asking for forgiveness?"

She paused, thinking about it. "Yes, I can ask for forgiveness."

Amy seemed tired. She had done much work. I took her hands and, looking into her eyes, said, "The work you are doing is good work. It took a lot of energy and courage, and you are doing an excellent job." She relaxed a bit more. We completed the session, scheduling another in a week.

When Amy returned, she had connected with her daughter on the East Coast. Her son and other daughter were coming to visit. She still felt anxious, but something significant had shifted. She was moving in the right direction; a path forward had opened.

We continued working on being at peace with life and being at peace with death. She said she needed to ask forgiveness of all her children. Elena said she would help Amy and her family.

I learned later from Elena that Amy successfully worked through the troubling issues with her family. A couple of months later, she passed away peacefully in her home, surrounded by her children and friend Elena. She had found peace and balance with her life and her death.

Discussion

When Elena came to me asking for help on behalf of her friend, I realized, first and foremost, I needed to help Amy find peace within herself. Second, I needed to respect Amy's values and wishes. I cannot make someone feel or believe something; that is never my intention. My intention is to help them feel their own feelings and honor those feelings that come from their deepest wisdom.

But how can I talk about deepest wisdom when the person is demented? In my opinion, these are two different, non-exclusive situations. Dementia has to do with the loss of ability to form new memories, to perform complex or simple tasks, and to care for oneself safely. Inner wisdom has to do with accessing a deep, inner knowing that does not depend on memory or physical health. It has facets and dimensions, like a hologram, which can be accessed and understood in various ways.

My responsibility is to bring wholeness to the client rather than do what the client asks for when they are conflicted and confused. In the case of Amy, it meant bringing her to the best possible state of being she could achieve and be. That means to be at peace with the moment, at peace with her life, at peace with life in general, and to be free of fear and anxiety about life or death.

When you are in the dark, if you sit quietly you often can discern a dim light you would not notice if you were moving about, seeking light. In other words, by thinking only of ending the darkness, you miss the light that is present. The work with Amy felt to me like being with her in a dark cave, and I was helping her to find that glimmer. The work we did allowed Amy to notice the darkness and appreciate the dim light she otherwise could not see. When she calmed down, she could stop feeling threatened by the darkness. She could see the glimmer of what she needed.

I did not hold the answers; I guided her to find them by holding the space for her so she could accept them and not be afraid. When she discovered her relationship with her children needed healing, she relaxed, her anxiety lightened, and I could sense the peace she experienced by her calmer breath, her facial relaxation, the tearing in her eyes.

Tearing is a sign of release and often a sign of relaxation. It is mediated by the vagus nerve, which is part of the parasympathetic nervous system. Similar signs include slowing down the breath, slowing the heart rate, salivating, burping, passing gas, and needing to urinate or to have a bowel movement. They are all signs of parasympathetic activation and release.

When someone is anxious and does not know why, there generally is a good reason, even if it does not appear to be logical. That reason is very specific for that person, which is why using drugs or self-medicating with alcohol or other substances often fails to resolve the problem. The person needs more drugs, more alcohol, new drugs, and the cycle continues. However, when one faces their fear and anxiety—by no means an easy task—one can expect to reduce and resolve them. A proficient guide, a skilled therapist, can provide the calm and confidence needed to complete the journey.

In his book *Many Deaths, One Life*, H. Brownell Wheeler, MD, FACS, talked about end of life and his experience as a surgeon caring for people facing death. As a bright physician trained to save lives, he did not understand how "extreme life-saving interventions could be perceived as a curse" by patients and their families. He was shocked to learn a person could prefer death over a life of misery. Only when he understood their suffering, pain, and other hardships—resulting from "heroic," expensive treatments—did he appreciate the meaning of "First Do No Harm." He changed his goal from life-saving interventions to delivering whatever served the patient's most desirable outcome, including dying with dignity, free from suffering.

EXERCISE: HARMONY MEDITATION
10-18 minutes

This meditation is beneficial when you are faced with a decision you are conflicted about. Thinking of the conflicting situation once the light moves up and down between the center of the brain and the center of the chest can bring insights and clarity to the situation.

Sit comfortably. Notice your breath.

Notice the right side of your face. As you inhale, allow the breath to fill the right side of your forehead. Repeat this two or three times, noticing how the breath can be directed to the right side of the forehead.

With the next inhale, allow the breath to move into your right eye. Repeat this one to two times.

With the next inhale, allow the breath to go into your right ear. Repeat this one to two times. Proceed to:

- breathe into your right cheek, one to two times;
- breathe into your right nostril, one to two times;
- inhale into the right side of your mouth, a few times;

- inhale into the right side of your chin, a few times; and
- inhale into the whole right side of your face.

With each part of your face, notice how it feels. How does it feel on the right compared to the left side of your face?

Now repeat the above steps with the left side of your face.

After you have completed the breathing with the left side of the face, focus on the midpoint between the right and left sides of your face, somewhere in the middle of the head, between the ears.

Next, proceed to repeat these steps with your focus on your chest, paying attention to the right chest:

- breathe into the right upper chest;
- breathe into the right middle chest;
- breathe into the right lower chest; and
- breathe into the whole right chest.

Repeat by breathing into the left chest.

Now focus on the connection between the right and the left parts of your chest, in the area of the heart.

Imagine a light at the midpoint in the head.

Imagine another light at the midpoint of the chest.

Imagine a connection between the two lights in the head and in the heart.

As you inhale, the light from the heart moves to the head. As you exhale, the light moves back to the heart. Repeat this a few minutes before letting go of the image and returning to natural breathing.

Notice how you feel.

Chapter 19: Tess and Maria

Two Cases of Phobias

*The thing you fear most has no power; your
fear of it is what has the power. Facing the
truth really will set you free.* – Oprah

CASE 1: TESS

Emetophobia is the fear of vomiting, including a fear of vomiting in public, a fear of seeing vomit, a fear of watching the action of vomiting, or a fear of being nauseated. It is common for emetophobics to be underweight or even anorexic, due to strict diets and restrictions they make for themselves. I had recently helped a young woman who wanted to become a nurse overcome her dread of vomiting, and I felt confident when Melanie called and asked if I dealt with children's phobias; her six-year-old daughter Tess had developed an intense fear of vomiting over the past six months. She experienced frequent abdominal pain and was afraid to eat. "I don't know what to do," Melanie said. "The situation is getting worse."

I assured Melanie I could help her daughter overcome her phobia easily and rapidly.

When she arrived with her mother, Tess looked composed and behaved in a mature, calm manner. Sitting in the armchair next to her mom, she looked at her mother inquisitively. Melanie said, "Tess has something she wants to give you." Tess handed me a page filled with her own handwriting. It read:

Food poisoning feelings:

• *scared*

• *bothered*

• *disgusted*

• *annoyed*

• *mindful*

• *unwanted*

• *not strong*

• *sad*

• *mad*

• *it comes and goes*

I learned Tess had been her normal self—an intelligent and sensitive girl—until the previous Thanksgiving. Her grandmother and grandfather were visiting for the holidays, and everyone got sick with a gastrointestinal flu, which entailed vomiting and other symptoms. Her grandfather became seriously ill and later died.

Since that episode, Tess felt scared and developed overwhelming, intense anxiety. She became preoccupied with frailty and illness and had obsessive thoughts that any food she encountered had not been safely prepared and would make her sick. Eating anything became difficult. She no longer wanted to go to parties or socialize when food was involved. She missed school on several occasions because of abdominal pain and feeling sick, episodes that increased in severity and frequency. Tess also was preoccupied with concerns about the safety of her father, a firefighter.

I asked her to tell me about that feeling. Pointing to her belly, she described a dark, jumbled black thing in her stomach, about the size of a large grapefruit.

I guided her through an integrative energy psychology process. Melanie also followed along with her daughter. After some time, I asked Tess if she noticed anything. She sighed and looked more relaxed. The grapefruit-sized shape in her stomach diminished: down to the size of a quarter, a pea, a thin piece of paper, and finally it disappeared. She no longer felt scared, bothered, disgusted, or annoyed. Tess now expressed wanting "to enjoy my whole life and like everything." She felt more confident and happy.

Melanie looked pleased, and yet I sensed she remained concerned. I observed Tess was also aware of her mother's uncertainty. I encouraged both mother and daughter to focus on the present feeling of confidence and comfort with foods, and I asked Melanie to follow up in a week for a session alone.

At the next session, Melanie informed me Tess continued doing so much better and appeared more relaxed and confident. She brought me a note from Tess. It listed her feelings:

- *happy*
- *sometimes scared*
- *sometimes nervous*
- *more confident*

Turning my attention to Melanie, I learned she had felt tension and anxiety since the original incident at Thanksgiving. She also felt helpless, unable to intervene or protect her daughter.

Although Tess had improved and no longer feared getting food poisoning, Melanie continued to worry. "What if Tess gets sick again or doesn't want to go to school? I don't know how to handle that. How can I promise nothing will ever make her sick again?"

As I helped Melanie release her own anxieties and feelings of helplessness, a memory from her childhood surfaced, eliciting these same feelings. At age six, as the result of a car accident, she suffered a concussion that required her to spend the night in the hospital. At the time, parents were not allowed to stay with their children, and she was alone throughout the night. The experience had terrified her, and she recalled the fear vividly. With guidance to process the trauma and those feelings, Melanie realized she was now an adult and in a different time, no longer a helpless little girl. The terror abated.

By the end of the session she felt relaxed and confident she could support Tess and could help her without having that anxious feeling. We agreed she and Tess would return in a month to complete the work and clear any fear or concern remaining.

One month later Tess brought me a note saying she felt:

• *scared - a little*

• *happy*

• *confident*

Melanie reported Tess enjoyed the foods she ate, except those prepared with garlic, especially pizza; then feelings of disgust and nausea recurred.

I did not have to explain what to do this time. I used Ask and Receive to treat Tess's aversion to garlic, as I would deal with an allergy. Within thirty minutes she felt fine with garlic in her pizza. Melanie called me a month later: Tess continued doing well and remained confident, secure, and happy. Melanie also felt more positive and relaxed.

Case 2: Maria

Maria, a forty-five-year-old mother and professional, came to me seeking help for an intense fear of flying (aerophobia). Just thinking about flying in an airplane caused severe anxiety, tight chest, sweaty palms, racing heart, and panting. For more than ten years, she had not traveled by plane to visit family or friends, though she realized her fear was irrational. Maria knew other people could fly safely, and she did not experience anxiety if her family flew. For herself, however, she could not overcome her phobia. Though she wanted to be with her family on vacations, if it involved air travel, she didn't go. She limited her vacations to car trips.

We began by discussing some of the most traumatic events in her life, including her experience, at age eleven, when her best friend's father died suddenly. A pilot, he died in a small-plane crash. Maria was devastated by her dear friend's grief and trauma, as well as her own loss of someone she respected and admired. She still felt sadness thinking about that memory.

I guided Maria to a peaceful place in her mind, where she felt safe and secure, and then slowly encouraged her to focus on her emotions about flying. As she did so, she described her chest tightening, her heart speeding up, her breathing becoming shallow and rapid, and feeling intense fear. While tapping on acupoints, we acknowledged these feelings and symptoms, as well as her sadness for her childhood experience.

Remembering that her fear of flying became more severe after her children were born, Maria realized she feared flying because she wanted to stay alive for her children. She had developed an unconscious belief that if she flew, she would orphan her children.

We cleared this belief, and she no longer felt anxiety and fear about flying. These feelings were replaced with a sense of anticipation and looking forward to seeing family and friends. Over the next few years, Maria flew several times and reported enjoying her travel experiences.

Discussion

There are many hypotheses for how and why phobias occur and resolve. I have used various techniques with different people, and they always resolved without difficulty. The longest it ever took me to help someone overcome a phobia was three sessions; the shortest was ten minutes with TFT. Accessing a childhood trauma is not necessary, but when it happens, the phobia resolves more rapidly. In these cases, Maria, Tess, and Melanie each recalled a single traumatic event that was involved.

Phobias are common. Twenty-five million Americans have aerophobia, or fear of flying. If the fear is due to a personal traumatic event in childhood, then treating everyone the same way, such as using anxiolytic drugs, will not address the individual trauma. Anxiolytics may result in some relief, but it will fail to address each individual's personal story. One size doesn't fit all. The doctor needs to be attuned to the patient's particular history and makeup. This is strikingly apparent in pharmacology, where different people react differently to the same drug. In hypertension, for example, some patients require stronger doses or additional drugs, because their blood pressure continues to rise. However, when the source of the anxiety is released, the blood pressure will normalize with lower doses or even without medications.

Since humans are not robots, they do not behave in an automatic way or respond in predetermined ways. The same trigger can create different responses in different individuals, so it is impossible to be certain what the response will be. Accepting this uncertainty allows for recognizing the uniqueness of each individual—and this clears the path for finding true solutions.

Exercise: Accessing love
5-10 minutes

This exercise was part of a meditation Rabbi David Zaslow used during prayer. It is similar to other practices to heal heart wounds and the neurolinguistic programming (NLP) technique for decreasing pain.

Sit comfortably. Put your attention on your breath. Think of someone you love. Notice where in your body love opens and flows freely. Enjoy this feeling for a few breaths. Release that image.

Next notice where in your body love is blocked. Allow yourself to sit with that part, with compassion, for a few breaths.

Now take the part where love is flowing freely and allow it to reach out to the part where love is blocked.

Repeat as necessary. Feel the love flow more freely.

Notice how you feel. Notice your breath.

In Closing

Making the Case for Alternative, Integrative Healing

*Perhaps part of the process of becoming
a clinician lies in learning to see
beyond the rules when the situation
requires it.* – Raphael Rush, MD

I OFTEN ASK people what was the most difficult part of the work
we did. The most common answer is, "Coming to see you."
Therefore, when someone walks through my door, I know they
have overcome a most difficult step, and I can begin our work
together with confidence, optimism, and compassion.

Why is it easier to take a pill than to summon from within
our innate capacity to heal? For many—as in my own case—the
answer lies with fear of the unknown, despair over past disap-
pointments, and simply being unaware of one's own powers and
strengths. It is my hope that the cases I've presented demonstrate
that health and well-being can be achieved, and that *you* are your
most effective ally and resource.

In medical school I learned that 85 percent of health problems are stress related, including heart disease, asthma, migraines, pain, inflammation, hypertension, diabetes, arthritis, cancer, obesity, autoimmune disease, allergies, and depression. Conventional medicine prescribes drugs or surgery to treat these conditions. Though the symptoms may be relieved, the origin of the problem remains—which as we now know, stems from childhood traumas and adverse experiences. In my work, often the most helpful part of the session is addressing the most difficult issue coming up in the moment. When we bring our focus to that and clear the root cause of the troubling feelings accompanying the problem, healing happens naturally and more easily.

I hope these pages have brought you a new paradigm for health and an understanding of how easy and possible healing can be. The magnitude of the problem doesn't really matter; how you address the *core* of the problem makes all the difference. Like a sailor's knot, your problem may look complicated and impregnable, but if you know the secret of untying it, you unravel it with ease.

Resources to help you are numerous; many more exist besides those I have mentioned. Search, explore, and be curious about what will work best for *you* to restore and renew your health. Don't be afraid. Learn to get in touch with your essence, and trust that part of you that knows—it has the power to heal.

Appendix A:
Anti-inflammatory Diet

An anti-inflammatory diet is one that sustains health and prevents illness, disease, and inflammation. A basic principle of an anti-inflammatory diet is to eat real food that has not been altered or processed, such as vegetables, fruits, nuts, and mushrooms. Other principles include:

- **Cook using simple methods:** steaming; pit- or earth-cooking, as is done in Hawaiian and Native American traditions; and quick stir-fry, as done in China.

- **Eat a colorful combination** of foods, such as

  » **greens and bitters:** swiss chard, collard greens, kale, lettuce, dandelion greens, mustard greens, beet greens; and herbs like cilantro, parsley, dill, chives, etc.;

  » **crucifers:** broccoli, cauliflower, cabbage, brussel sprouts, etc.;

  » **roots:** carrots, parsnip, daikon, beets, rutabaga, radish, yams, potato, celery root;

  » **plant fruits:** cucumbers, tomatoes, peppers, zucchini, squashes; and tree fruits: citrus, apples, pears, mangoes, berries, papayas, pineapples; and

  » **other whole foods:** ginger, turmeric, horseradish, onions, garlic, tea, and other herbs.

- **Eat local** fresh fruits, vegetables, and produce.

- **Eat fermented foods** with healthy probiotics, such as sauerkraut, pickled daikon, kombucha, yogurt, and buttermilk. Many of these are easy to make at home.

- **Eat seasonal**: in spring and summer, more greens, fruits, and vegetables; in winter and fall, more fat, soups, stews, and warming foods.

- **Eat organic** (or wild) when possible, especially foods that concentrate toxins, such as mushrooms, seaweed, herbs, and dirty-dozen foods (that have high levels of pesticides and should be avoided if not organic), which include juices and dried foods, such as apples, pears, peaches, berries, lettuce and leafy greens, nectarines, celery, cherries, peppers, tomatoes, grapes, and potatoes.

- **Eat least-contaminated foods** that contain smaller amounts of pesticides and are relatively safe to consume when not organic: onions, avocado, pineapples, mango, asparagus, sweet peas (frozen), kiwi, bananas, cabbage, and broccoli.

Just as important as consuming wholesome foods is avoiding processed foods that are inflammatory. Commonly processed foods are hydrogenated fats, trans fats, refined sugar, refined salt, fructose, high-fructose corn syrup, rice syrup, concentrated apple juice or any concentrated or adulterated (with added concentrates) fruit juice, modified food starch, white flour, alcohol, artificial flavors, artificial color, preservatives, words you can't pronounce or understand, fortified foods (which have been processed and stripped of their nutrients in the processing so they have to be "fortified" to replenish some of those nutrients), and genetically modified foods (corn, wheat, canola, soy).

- **Avoid or minimize meats**, especially those not grass-fed and finished. If you eat meats or fowl, then eat them sparingly and choose grass-fed or pastured fowl (and eggs) that have been cared for and humanely treated.

- **Consume pasture-raised eggs** or those from local, small-family farms where chickens are free to roam and eat insects and plants.

- **Avoid GMO foods.** These are foods genetically modified to resist pests by incorporating toxins against those pests. These toxins are often toxic to humans, as well.

- **Minimize casein in dairy products**: casein, a milk protein, is high in cow milk, lower in goat milk, lowest in sheep milk—almost as low as human breast milk. Casein consumption is correlated with increased diabetes incidence and hypertension.

- **Avoid homogenized milk,** as it overwhelms the human digestive system and causes increased VLDL (very low density lipoprotein—bad cholesterol) and prevents proper fat metabolism. Non-homogenized whole milk, also called *cream top,* where the cream (fat) is separated from the milk, is available and is easier to digest. If homogenized, then skim milk having less fat will be less likely to overpower your digestion of fats.

- **Consume essential fats**: DHA—an important fat for the maintenance of brain function, BRNF (brain-derived neurotropic factor), and prevention of changes leading to degenerative processes such as Alzheimer's disease—can be found in sardines, salmon, caviar, and brain and organ meat. Omega-3 fatty acids also are found in sardines, salmon, pastured eggs, caviar, and krill.

- Avoid large, cold-water fish, which often are contaminated with mercury and PCBs, such as swordfish, tuna, and king salmon.

- Use caution with farm-raised fish, which often are exposed to antibiotics. Their feeding is not a natural marine diet and may include toxins and chemicals.

These are general guidelines. Each individual may respond differently to certain foods, depending on whether they have allergies or sensitivities to that particular food. When an individual has a sensitivity or allergy, then the food can be inflammatory. This is a condition that can be treated energetically. This is in contrast to foods that contain toxins such as aflatoxin or pesticides, which must be avoided and cannot be made safe.

Appendix B: Diagrams of Poses

1. Eyebrow points (2: one left and one right).
2. Side of eye or outer eye points (2: from outer eye to edge of cheekbone).
3. Eye or under eye point (2: both eyes).
4. Under nose point (1).
5. Under lip point (1).
6. Collarbone points (2: one left and one right): just under collarbone, one inch below collarbone and one inch to the side of the sternum (breast bone).
7. Under arm points (2: one left and one right): four finger-widths below armpit, in the middle of the side of the chest (mid-axillary line).
8. Liver points (2: one left and one right): over middle of the last rib, aligned with the nipple.

9. KC (Karate Chop) (2: one left and one right): area on the side of the hand between the bones (metacarpals) leading to the little finger and the wrist.

10. Gamut: area on the back of the hand between the bones (metacarpals) leading to the little finger and ring finger.

11. NLR: Neurolymphatic reflex points (2: the left is much more useful than the right).

TFT/EFT
ACUPOINTS

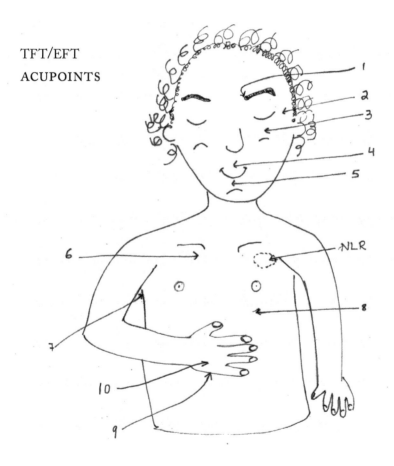

Collarbone breathing exercise

1. Start by placing the index finger and the middle finger on the collarbone point. (Fig. A1)

2. As you tap on the gamut point with the fingers of your other hand, take a full breath in. (Fig. A2)

3. Keep tapping as you hold your breath to the count of 7 taps. (Fig. A2)

4. Breathe halfway out (empty your lungs halfway). (Fig. A2)

5. Hold your breath for 7 taps. (Fig. A2)

6. Breathe out the rest of the breath. (Fig. A2)

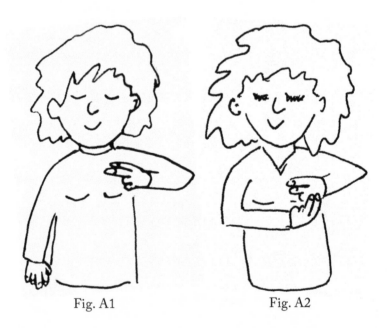

Fig. A1   Fig. A2

7. Hold your breath as you tap 7 times. (Fig. A2)

8. Breathe halfway in (fill your lungs halfway). Again hold your breath as you tap 7 times. (Fig. A2)

9. Again hold your breath as you tap 7 times. (Fig. A2)

10. Take a natural breath. (Fig. A2)

Then move your fingers to the other side of the chest on the collarbone point (Fig. A3), and continue steps 2 through 10, above.

Now make a fist with your thumb inside your folded fingers, and place the knuckle on the collarbone point (Fig. B1)

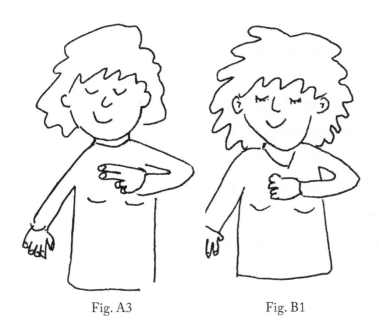

Fig. A3   Fig. B1

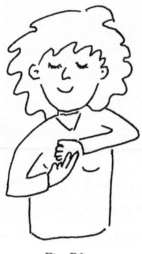

Fig. B2

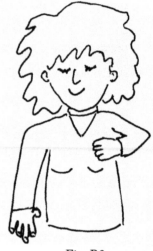

Fig. B3

Repeat the breathing-and-holding-breath sequence while tapping, as above (steps 2-10), until you take a natural breath. (Fig. B2)

Move your fist to the other collarbone point, placing the knuckle on the collarbone point. (Fig. B3)

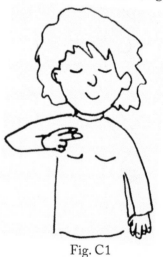

Repeat the breathing-and-holding-breath sequence while tapping, as above (steps 2-10), until you take a natural breath.

Now you're ready to repeat sequence 1-10, starting with the other hand. (Fig. C1)

Fig. C1

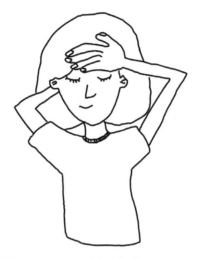

Fronto-occipital hold: front view

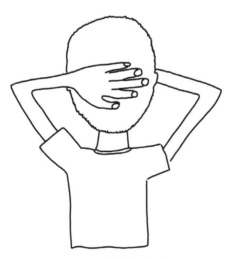

Fronto-occipital hold: back view

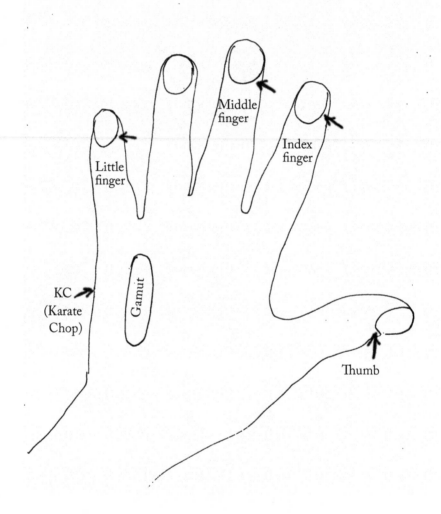

Appendix C: Glossary

Acupuncture. This ancient Chinese medical practice manipulates the flow of energy, or *Qi* (pronounced *chee*), in the body and organs by inserting needles in specific points on the body to evoke a physiological healing response. It has been proven to be effective with diminishing pain, allergic symptoms, and other disease conditions. Acupuncturists receive four years of training and earn a DOM, doctor of Oriental Medicine, degree. There are several specialties that use natural herbs and supplements to treat symptoms and tonify or sedate organs.

Ask and Receive (A&R). A&R was developed in 2009 by Sandi Radomski, a naturopathic physician and social worker who specializes in eliminating allergies and other physical maladies, and her colleague, Tom Altaffer, a social worker. It is a simple and powerful technique and can be used alone or in combination with other energy modalities. Find out more about A&R at http://askandreceive.org.

Be Set Free Fast (BSFF) was developed by Larry Nims in the 1980s. BSFF programs the subconscious mind to dissolve negative beliefs, feelings, or thoughts and instill desirable feelings and thoughts by using a shortcut to the subconscious in the form of a cue. See http://www.besetfree.com.

Centering. Being centered allows one to feel grounded and balanced. Several practices allow for centering: Qi Gong, yoga, slow deep breathing, ujjayi breathing, and walking barefoot on the earth, to name a few. When one is centered, one's mind is clearer, more at ease, and insights are more likely to happen. Things that unbalance and prevent centering are lack of sleep, feeling stressed, dehydration, emotional triggers, certain drugs, electromagnetic fields (EMFs), toxic substances, allergens, and physical ailments.

Core Transformation. An elegant technique developed by Connierae Andreas, PhD, to help individuals overcome emotional, physical, and spiritual difficulties and achieve a deep level of healing. Through this process, one often attains higher states of consciousness and well-being. http://www.coretransformation.org.

Diet. What is in the foods and drinks we ingest is a central question to health. In this book, "diet" does not refer to a particular regimen or whether to avoid certain foods or to adhere to a certain caloric content.

Emotional Freedom Technique (EFT). This energy psychology technique, based on Thought Field Therapy (TFT), was developed by Gary Craig. EFT is performed by tapping on all the acupuncture points on the face and body, as well as repeating key phrases and reciting relevant words or challenging statements to access the unconscious mind. It is simple to use and, like TFT, it is common to be able to clear phobias and reduce acute or even chronic pain. Emofree.com and energypsych.org.

Energy psychology (EP) is defined by the Association for Comprehensive Energy Psychology (ACEP) as a collection of mind-body approaches for understanding and improving human functioning. EP focuses on the relationship between thoughts, emotions, sensations, behaviors, and known bioenergy systems (such as meridians and the biofield). For more information and to find a list of practitioners, see http://www.energypsych.org/.

Eye Movement Desensitization and Reprocessing (EMDR). A psychotherapeutic method introduced in the 1980s by Francine Shapiro, PhD, which entails activating both sides of the brain and accessing memories, addressing the effects of those memories, and processing memories and feelings to bring peace and neutrality to the individual. It has been effective for treating PTSD, depression, anxiety, and other conditions. See http://www.emdr.com and http://parnellemdr.com.

Focusing technique was developed in the 1970s by Gene Gendlin while doing postdoctoral research on effective therapies. He audiotaped hundreds of therapy sessions and followed the patients for six months. He discovered that he could predict, with 96 percent accuracy, which patients were going to have beneficial outcomes by listening to fifteen minutes of their first or second session. He created a simple technique with six steps to allow and facilitate this process. Research shows that using the first step alone—clearing a space—can improve the quality of life in breast cancer survivors. Dr. Davie is certified as a Focusing Trainer and uses this technique often as the basis of successful therapy. http://www.focusing.org.

Food supplements. For medicinal and health reasons, supplemental nutrition with vitamins, herbs, and minerals are used.

Fronto-occipital (FO) **hold.** A position where the hands hold the head, with one palm on the forehead and the other on the occiput. This position has been used in many modalities—including craniosacral, energy psychology, healing from the body level up (HBLU), and other indigenous and energy techniques—to help calm and balance the individual. (See the diagram, pages 178-179.)

Functional medicine is a new specialty of medicine that looks at the whole individual and tries to determine the cause of the symptom and correct it with various approaches including supplements, environmental factors, nutrition, exercise, massage, and other alternative and conventional modalities. https://www.ifm.org/functional-medicine/.

Guided imagery/Visualization is a technique that helps a person imagine and visualize specific scenes to effect specific goals. It may be considered a form of hypnosis and has been used for relaxation; relief of allergies, asthma, and pain; decreasing inflammation; boosting the immune system; preparing for surgery; and even abating cancer.

Healing from the body level up (HBLU™) is a holistic psychotherapy system to clear mental, emotional, physical, and spiritual blocks to success. Developed by Judith A. Swack, PhD, HBLU integrates her original research with biomedical science, psychology, spirituality, applied kinesiology, hypnosis, Neurolinguistic Programming, and other energy psychology techniques. Learn more at http://www.hblu.org.

Healing Touch. See Therapeutic Touch (TT).

HeartMath. A research-backed technology utilizing the body's natural rhythms and science to improve well-being. It has been proven to alleviate anxiety, depression, and stress responses. Learn more at http://www.heartmath.com.

Heart pose. Both hands are held on the heart, with one palm on the chest and the other palm on top of that hand.

Heart Rate Variability (HRV) is the change in heart rate from heartbeat to heartbeat, depending on the respiratory cycle. A higher variability of the heart rate is correlated with longevity and well-being.

Holographic Memory Resolution (HMR). Developed by Brendt Baum, an archeologist, minister, and social worker, this effective tool helps people heal from physical and emotional issues. http://www.healingdimensions.com/index.html.

Ho'oponopono. A Hawaiian healing practice using forgiveness and love, it involves saying and/or repeating four statements:
I am sorry.
Please forgive me.
Thank you.
I love you.

Hypnosis. According to the American Psychological Association, hypnosis is a procedure during which a health professional or researcher suggests, while treating someone, that he or she experience changes in sensations, perceptions, thoughts, or behavior. Clinical hypnosis is successfully used for many conditions, including pain, inflammation, and various physical and emotional conditions. The Milton Erickson Foundation is a good resource: https://www.erickson-foundation.org/.

Intentions and statements of goals. In Dr. Davie's practice, sessions often begin with an intention that integrates a prayer, statements from the client's own words, her own words, Soul Retrieval, HBLU, and other energy psychology techniques to facilitate the mindset for the healing to occur safely and with ease.

Mind-body healing. Healing that encompasses multiple dimensions and feels congruent with the whole person: physically, emotionally, mentally, and spiritually.

Neurolinguistic Programming (NLP) is a form of therapy developed by Richard Bandler and John Grinder. It uses language patterns to communicate with the meaning of the unconscious beliefs and address them. A skilled therapist can help with anxiety, phobias, and many psychological issues. http://www.nlpoftherockies.com.

Orthomolecular medicine. A term coined by Nobel laureate Linus Pauling. The Foundation of Orthomolecular Medicine states: "The goal of orthomolecular medicine is to restore the body's optimal environment by correcting imbalances or deficiencies based on individual biochemistry by using natural substances such as vitamins, minerals, trace elements, and amino acids." http://www.faim.org and http://www.orthomolecular.org.

Qi Gong is an ancient, holistic Chinese practice for health and wellness. It involves coordinated movements and meditations, with attention on the breath, sounds, balance, stillness, and flowing movements to support the life force and enhance well-being. It is the basis for martial arts such as Tai Chi and Karate. Medical Qi Gong is a specialized form of Qi Gong to heal physical and emotional problems. Practicing Qi Gong regularly is safe and often improves health, balance, awareness, and relaxation.

Reconnective Healing is an energetic healing therapy discovered and introduced by a chiropractor, Eric Pearl. While working on his patients, he discovered that some people seemed to heal miraculously. He investigated these results and developed this healing method, which he explains to be an act of "God/Love/Light/Source." He teaches the technique all over the world. See https://www.thereconnection.com.

Reiki is an ancient Japanese spiritual healing modality using the laying of hands to facilitate healing from various physical and emotional conditions. Receiving a Reiki treatment from a skilled practitioner often helps with relaxation, relieves pain and discomfort, improves sleep, and imparts many other benefits. Prominent cancer centers, such as Dana Farber Cancer Institute of Boston, recommend Reiki to their patients as an adjunct to medical treatment. The Dana Farber Cancer Institute states: "Reiki is a simple, natural, and safe method of spiritual healing and self-improvement that most everyone can benefit from. It has been found to be effective in helping every known illness, including cancer."

Relaxation is defined as being free from anxiety or tension. When a person is relaxed, breaths are slow, deep, long, and comfortable. Heart rate is slower, muscles are relaxed, and the person feels calm and tranquil.

Soul Detective. An energy psychology modality developed by Dr. Barbara Stone to find the hidden origins of mental and emotional distress. The step-by-step protocols she developed cover a broad range of topics including ancestral wounds, helping earthbound spirits cross to the light, and releasing detrimental energies. Learn more at http://www.Souldetective.net.

Subjective Units of Discomfort/Distress (SUDS) or **Disturbance Scale.** This is a scale to help determine the intensity of an emotion or sensation—such as pain, anger, anxiety—and to determine the effect of a therapeutic intervention on the symptom. It usually ranges from one, or zero, to ten. For children, it is common to use smiley/frowny faces or sizes such as "big," with arms open wide, and "small," like a tiny point. Dr. Davie uses the zero-to-ten scale.

Tai Chi is a graceful, ancient Chinese martial art, commonly used as a non-competitive, low-impact practice with flowing movements that improve awareness, alertness, balance, strength, and breathing. It has been highly recommended for stress reduction and to improve balance in the elderly.

Therapeutic Touch (TT). An evidence-based, holistic therapy developed by Professor Dolores Krieger, PhD, RN and Dona Kunz, a natural healer. Scientific research supports its benefits for pain relief, cancer, inflammation, and numerous other conditions.

There are over 100,000 TT practitioners in the USA. http://thera-peutictouch.org.

Thought Field Therapy (TFT) was pioneered in the 1980s by Roger Callahan, PhD, a psychologist. Using his knowledge of kinesiology, developed by Dr. George Goodheart, and traditional acupuncture meridians, he discovered how to rapidly release stuck emotions such as anger, depression, phobias, and anxiety by using specific treatment algorithms. TFT is the first energy psychology modality to receive the designation of Evidence-based Therapy by the National Registry of Evidence-based Procedures and Practices (NREPP). http://www.rogercallahan.com, http://www.thought-fieldtherapy.net, and several others.

Visualization. See Guided imagery, above.

Appendix D: Recommended Resources

BOOKS

Andreas, Connierae, and Andreas, Tamara. 1994. *Core Transformation*. Moab, UT: Real People Press.

Arenson, Gloria. 2001. *Five Simple Steps to Emotional Healing*. New York: Simon and Schuster.

Bandler, Richard, and Grinder, John. 1979. *Frogs into Princes: Neurolinguistic Programming*. Moab, UT: Real People Press.

Bengston, William, with Fraser, Sylvia. 2010. *Chasing the Cure*. Toronto: Key Porter Books.

Bertherat, Therese, and Bernstein, Carol. 1989. *The Body Has Its Reasons: Self-Awareness through Conscious Movement*. Rochester, VT: Healing Arts Press.

Borysenko, Joan. 1993. *Fire in the Soul*. New York: Warner Books.

Braden, Gregg. 2014. *Resilience from the Heart: The Power to Thrive in Life's Extremes*. Hay House, Inc.

Brawley, Otis W., and Goldberg, Paul. 2012. *How We Do Harm: A Doctor Breaks Rank about Being Sick in America*. NY: Macmillan.

> *A book by a conscientious oncologist reporting on how conflict of interest and pharmaceutical involvement affect the quality of care for cancer patients.*

Bray, Robert. 2008. *No Open Wounds—Heal Traumatic Stress NOW*. Robertson Publishing.

A very good book about TFT, with algorithms and with examples and case studies.

Brockman, Howard. 2006. *Dynamic Energetic Healing: Integrating Core Shamanic Practices with Energy Psychology Applications and Process Work Principles.* Salem, OR: Columbia Press, LLC.

Burk, Larry. 2012. *Let Magic Happen: Adventures in Healing with a Holistic Radiologist.* Healing Imagery Press.

Campbell, T. Colin, and Campbell, Thomas II. 2005. *The China Study.* Dallas, TX: BenBella Books.

In their book, Cornell University scientists present international research correlating diet, nutrition, and health.

Casarjian, Robin. 1992. *Forgiveness: A Bold Choice for a Peaceful Heart.* NY: Bantam.

A good introduction to and basic principles of forgiveness.

Chopra, Deepak. 1989. *Ageless Bodies, Timeless Minds.* NY: Crown Publishing Group.

Chopra, Deepak. 1989. *Quantum Healing.* NY: Bantam Books.

Connolly, Suzanne M. 2004. *Thought Field Therapy.* Sedona, AZ: George Tyrrell Press.

Cousens, Gabriel. 2013. *There Is a Cure for Diabetes: The 21-Day+ Holistic Recovery Program.* Berkeley, CA: North Atlantic Books.

This book, written by a physician, researcher, and scholar, has a lot of information on the bad effects of sugar on the body and how to cure diabetes. In my opinion, because sugar is inflammatory and has many adverse effects on the body, the information applies to autoimmune disease, inflammatory conditions, and overall well-being. The diet, somewhat challenging for the average person, has much to offer in terms of possibilities and choices.

Craig, Gary. 2008. *The EFT Manual.* Santa Rosa, CA: Energy Psychology Press.

Diamond, John. 1979. *Your Body Doesn't Lie: Unlock the Power of Your Natural Energy!* NY: Warner Books.

Dossey, Larry. 1993. *Healing Words: The Power of Prayer and the Practice of Medicine.* San Francisco: Harper San Francisco.

Dossey, Larry. 2007. *The Extraordinary Healing Power of Ordinary Things: Fourteen Natural Steps to Health and Happiness.* PA: Harmony (reprint edition).

Ecker, Bruce, et al. 2012. *Unlocking the Emotional Brain: Eliminating Symptoms at Their Roots Using Memory Reconsolidation.* NY: Routledge.

Eden, Donna. 2008. *Energy Medicine.* NY: Jeremy P. Tarcher/Penguin.

Elliott, Stephen. 2005. *The New Science of Breath: Coherent Breathing for Autonomic Nervous System Health and Well-being.* Allen, TX: Coherence Press.

Feinstein, David, Eden, Donna, and Craig, Gary. 2005. *The Promise of Energy Psychology.* NY: Jeremy P. Tarcher/Penguin.

Foundation for Inner Peace. 1976. *A Course in Miracles.* Foundation for Inner Peace.

Fuhrman, Joel. 2012. *The End of Diabetes: The Eat to Live Plan to Prevent and Reverse Diabetes*. NY: Harper One.

> *Dr. Fuhrman explains facts about diabetes and its treatment with dietary and lifestyle changes. This program can be applied to many other health conditions, specifically those with inflammation.*

Gawande, Atul. 2014. *Being Mortal*. NY: Metropolitan Books.

Gendlin, Eugene. 1981. *Focusing*. New York: New Bantam Books.

Gold, Rabbi Sheffa. 2006. *Torah Journeys: The Inner Path to the Promised Land*. NJ: Ben Yehuda Press.

> *The author teaches a spiritual practice that helps us listen with our hearts to the inner wisdom that comes when we see prayers as a mirror. Guided meditations reveal the alchemy of this practice and demonstrate how to transform some of the deepest pain into positive emotions.*

Grossbart, Ted, and Sherman, Carl. 1992. *Skin Deep: A Mind/Body Program for Healthy Skin*. Health Press (revised edition).

Hanson, Rick. 2013. *Hardwiring Happiness: The New Brain Science of Contentment, Calm, and Confidence*. NY: Harmony Books.

> *Another book that shows you a simple technique on how you can tap into positive experiences to heal negative feelings.*

Hawkins, David R. 2009. *Healing and Recovery*. Hay House, Inc.

Hawkins, David R. 2001. *The Eye of the I*. Hay House, Inc.

Hawkins, David R. 1995. *Power vs. Force*. Hay House, Inc.

Hay, Louise L. 2004. *You Can Heal Your Life*. Hay House, Inc.

Huddleston, Peggy. 1996. *Prepare for Surgery and Heal Faster*. Cambridge, MA: Angel River Press.

Jackson, Paul. 2014. *Ho'oponopono Secrets: Four Phrases to Change the World, One Love to Bind Them*. Paul Jackson.

> *The essence and true meaning of practicing love and forgiveness.*

Jampolsky, Gerald. 2009. *Love Is Letting Go of Fear*. NY: Celestial Arts, a division of Random House.

Kabat-Zinn, John. 2005. *Wherever You Go There You Are: Mindfulness Meditation in Everyday Life*. NY: Hachette.

Krieger, Dolores. 1993. *Accepting Your Power to Heal: The Personal Practice of Therapeutic Touch*. Santa Fe, NM: Bear & Co.

Lewis, Byron, and Pucelik, Frank. 2012. *Magic of NLP Demystified: A Pragmatic Guide to Communications and Change*. NY: Crown House Pub. Ltd.

Lown, Bernard. 1996. *The Lost Art of Healing*. NY: Ballantine Books.

> *A prominent Harvard cardiologist recounts some of his thoughts and experiences with his patients with heart disease.*

Mundy, William L. 1993. *Curing Allergy with Visual Imagery*. East Canaan, CT: Safe Goods Publishing.

Myss, Carolyn. 1996. *Anatomy of the Spirit*. NY: Three Rivers Press.

Northrop, Christiane. 1998. *Women's Bodies, Women's Wisdom*. NY: Bantam Books.

Ogden, Pat. 2015. *Sensorimotor Psychotherapy: Interventions for Trauma and Attachment*. NY: W. W. Norton and Co.

Ogden, Pat. 2006. *Trauma and the Body: A Sensorimotor Approach to Psychotherapy* (Norton Series on Interpersonal Neurobiology). NY: W. W. Norton and Co.

Ornish, Dean. 1990. *Reversing Heart Disease*. NY: Ivy Books.

Pearl, Eric. 2001. *The Reconnection: Heal Others, Heal Yourself*. Hay House, Inc.

Perry, Bruce, and Szalavitz, Maia. 2017. *The Boy Who Was Raised as a Dog and Other Stories from a Child Psychiatrist's Notebook: What Traumatized Children Can Teach Us about Loss, Love, and Healing*. NY: Basic Books.

> *A remarkable book about the neurological and psychological effects of childhood tragedies and the potential for the healing and recovery of traumatized children.*

Rosen, Sidney. 1982. *My Voice Will Go with You: The Teaching Tales of Milton H. Erickson*. NY: W. W. Norton & Co.

Segal, Inna. 2007. *The Secret Language of Your Body*. Australia: Blue Angel Gallery.

Siegel, Daniel. 2010. *Mindsight: the New Science of Personal Transformation*. NY: Bantam Books.

> *This book explains the neuroscience of relationships and how to cultivate successful relationships.*

Stone, Barbara. 2008. *Invisible Roots*. Santa Rosa, CA: Energy Psychology Press.

> *Dr. Stone takes past-life regression to a new level and recounts her clinical experience of yet another powerful way for healing.*

van der Kolk, Bessel. 2015. *The Body Keeps the Score*. NY: Penguin.

> *Best-selling author and trauma specialist sheds light on healing from trauma*

Weiser-Cornell, Ann. 1996. *The Power of Focusing: A Practical Guide to Emotional Self-healing*. New Harbinger Publications.

Wheeler, H. Brownell. 2014. *One Life, Many Deaths: A Surgeon's Stories*. Meredith Winter Press.

Williams, Louisa. 2011. *Radical Medicine*. Rochester, VT: Healing Arts Press.

> *A textbook of health issues, with emphasis on current controversies in medicine and dentistry.*

Zieg, Jeffrey. 1980. *A Teaching Seminar with Milton H. Erickson*. NY: Brunner-Routledge.

Zeig, Jeffrey, and Gilligan, Stephen, eds. 1990. *Brief Therapy: Myths, Methods and Metaphors*. NY: Brunner Mazel.

Articles

Anda, R., Williamson, D., Jones, D., et al. 1993. "Depressed Affect, Hopelessness, and the Risk of Ischemic Heart Disease in a Cohort of U.S. Adults." *Epidemiology* 4 (July): 285–294.

Bengston, W. and Krinsley, D. 2000. "The Effect of the 'Laying-on of Hands' on Transplanted Breast Cancer in Mice." *Journal of Scientific Exploration* 14: 353-364.

Bengston, W. and Moga, M. 2007. "Resonance, Placebo Effects, and Type II Errors: Some Implications from Healing Research for Experimental Methods." *The Journal of Alternative and Complementary Medicine* 13: 317-327.

Bengston, W. 2007. Commentary: "A Method Used to Train Skeptical Volunteers to Heal in an Experimental Setting." *The Journal of Alternative and Complementary Medicine* 13: 329-331.

Bishop, K. S., and Ferguson, L. R. 2015. "The Interaction between Epigenetics, Nutrition and the Development of Cancer." *Nutrients* no. 7 (2): 922-947. https://doi/10.3390/nu7020922.

Borger, N., van der Meere, J., et al. 1999. "Heart Rate Variability and Sustained Attention in ADHD Children." *Journal of Abnormal Child Psychology* 27: 25-33.

Chajès, V. and Romieu, I. 2014. "Nutrition and Breast Cancer." *Maturitis* 77, no. 1: 7-11. https://doi/10.1016/j.maturitas.2013.10.004.

Carney, R. M., Saunders, R. D., et al. 1995. "Association of Depression with Reduced Heart Rate Variability In Coronary Artery Disease." *American Journal of Cardiology* 76: 562-565.

Chambliss, D. L., Sanderson, et al. 1996. "An update on Empirically Validated Therapies." *The Clinical Psychologist* 49: 5-18.

Chapman, L. F., et al. 1959. "Changes in Tissue Vulnerability During Hypnotic Suggestion." *Journal of Psychosomatic Research* 4: 99-105.

Cohen, H., Kotler, M., et al. 1998. "Analysis of Heart Rate Variability in Posttraumatic Stress Disorder Patients in Response to a Trauma-related Reminder." *Biological Psychiatry* 44 (10): 1054-1059.

Connolly, S. M., and Sakai, C. 2011. "Brief Trauma Symptom Intervention with Rwandan Genocide Survivors Using Thought Field Therapy." *International Journal of Emergency Mental Health* 13(3): 161-172. https://www.ncbi.nlm.nih.gov/pubmed/22708146.

Connolly, S. M., Roe-Sepowitz, D., Sakai, C., et al. 2013. "Utilizing Community Resources to Treat PTSD: A Randomized Controlled Trial Using Thought Field Therapy." *African Journal of Traumatic Stress* 3 (1): 24-32. http://www.petercaldermanfoundation.org/wp-content/uploads/2014/04/AJTS_V1N5smallpdf.com.pdf.

Dreaper, R. 1978. "Recalcitrant Warts on the Hand Cured by Hypnosis." *The Practitioner* 22: 305-310.

Han, B., et al. for the ALLHAT Collaborative Research Group. 2017. "Effect of Statin Treatment vs. Usual Care on Primary Cardiovascular Prevention among Older Adults." The ALLHAT-LLT Randomized Clinical Trial, published in *JAMA Internal Medicine* 177 (7): 955-965. https://doi:10.1001/jamainternmed.2017.1442.

Cholesterol-lowering drugs for primary prevention is of no benefit to elderly.

Felitti, V. J., Anda, R. F., et al. 1998. "Relationship of Childhood Abuse and Household Dysfunction to Many of the Leading Causes of Death in Adults: The Adverse Childhood Experiences

(ACE) Study." *American Journal of Preventive Medicine* 14, no. 4: 245-258. https://doi.org/10.1016/S0749-3797(98)00017-8.

> *This is a landmark study that proves beyond any doubt that adult disease is directly related to traumas in childhood. There are several presentations and lectures by Dr. Felitti available on YouTube about this research and the significance of its findings.*

Felitti, V. J. 2010. "Obesity: Problem, Solution, or Both?" *The Permanente Journal* 14(1): 24–30. https://www.ncbi.nlm.nih.gov/pmc/articles/PMC2912711/.

Felitti, V. J. 2015. "The Relationship of Adverse Childhood Experiences to PTSD, Depression, Poly-drug Use and Suicide Attempt in Reservation-based Native American Adolescents and Young Adults." *American Journal of Community Psychology* 55, no. 3-4: 411-421. https://doi.org/10.1007/s10464-015-9721-3.

Foo, S. Y., Heller, E. R., et al. 2009. "Vascular Effects of a Low-carbohydrate High-protein Diet." *Proceedings of the National Academy of Sciences.* 106, 15: 418-15,423.

Gilbert, L. K., et al. 2015. "Childhood Adversity and Adult Chronic Disease: An Update from Ten States and the District of Columbia." *American Journal of Preventive Medicine* 48, no. 3: 345–349. http://dx.doi.org/10.1016/j.amepre.2014.09.006.

> *This larger-scale ACE study with greater diversity included 50,000 participants in different geographic locations and confirmed the findings of Vincent Felitti's earlier study.*

Leaf, A. 1990. "Cardiovascular Effects of Fish Oils: Beyond the Platelet." *Circulation* 82: 624-628.

McCraty, R., Atkinson, M., et al. 1995. "The Effects of Emotions on Short-term Power Spectrum Analysis of Heart Rate Variability." *American Journal of Cardiology* 76: 1,089-1,093.

McDowell, M. 1949. "Juvenile Warts Removed with the Aid of Hypnotic Suggestion." *Bulletin of the Menninger Clinic* 13: 124-126.

Middleton, H. C., and Ashby, M. 1995. "Clinical Recovery from Panic Disorder Is Associated with Evidence of Changes in Cardiovascular Regulation." *Acta Psychiatrica Scandinavica* 1: 108-113.

Miller, Lisa, ed. 2012. "Spirituality, Connection, and Healing with Intent: Some Reflections on Cancer Experiments on Laboratory Mice," in *Oxford Handbook of Spirituality and Psychology*. Oxford University Press.

Miranda, S. P. 2017. "Learning to drive: Early Exposure to End-of-Life Conversations in Medical Training." *New England Journal of Medicine* 376, no. 5: 413-414.

Motoyama, H. 1993. "Energy Fields of the Organism." *Life Physics* 2 (1): 1-3.

Ornish, D., Scherwitz, L. W., Billings, J. H., et al. 1998. "Intensive Lifestyle Changes for Reversal of Coronary Heart Disease." *JAMA* 280: 2001-2007.

Ornish, D., et al. 1990. Can Lifestyle Changes Reverse Coronary Heart Disease? The Lifestyle Heart Trial." *The Lancet* vol. 336, no. 8708: 129–133.

Ray, Wayne, et al. 2009. "Atypical Antipsychotic Drugs and the Risk of Cardiac Death." *New England Journal of Medicine* 360: 225-235. http://dx.doi.org/10.1056/NEJMoa0806994.

Schoen, M., and Nowack, K. 2013. "Reconditioning the Stress Response with Hypnosis CD Reduces the Inflammatory Cytokine IL6 and Influences Resilience." *Complementary Therapies in Clinical Practice* 19 (2): 83-8.

Simpkin, A., and Schwartzstein, R. M. 2016. "Tolerating Uncertainty: the Next Medical Revolution? *New England Journal of Medicine* 375: 1713-1715. http://www.nejm.org/doi.org/full/10.1056/NEJMp1606402#t=article.

Sinclair-Gieben, A. H., and Chalmers, D. 1959. "Evaluation of Treatment of Warts by Hypnosis." *The Lancet* 10/3: 480-482.

Surman, O. S., et al. 1973. "Hypnosis in the Treatment of Warts." *Archives of General Psychiatry* 28: 439-441.

Tabatabaee A., et al. 2016. "Effect of Therapeutic Touch in Patients with Cancer: A Literature Review." *Med. Arch.* 70 http://dx.10.5455/medarh.2016.70.142-147.

Tasini, M. F., and Hackett, T. P. 1977. "Hypnosis in the Treatment of Warts in Immunodeficient Children." *American Journal of Clinical Hypnosis* 19: 152-154.

Teegarden, D., Romieu, I., and Lelièvre, S. A. 2012. "Redefining the Impact of Nutrition on Breast Cancer Incidence: Is Epigenetics Involved?" *Nutrition Research Reviews* 25, no. 1: 68-95. http://dx.10.1017/S0954422411000199.

Toker, S., et al. 2005. "The Association between Burnout, Depression, Anxiety, and Inflammation Biomarkers: C-Reactive Protein and Fibrinogen in Men and Women." *Journal of Occupational Health Psychology* 344-362. http://dx.10.1037/1076-8998.10.4.344.

von Känel, R., Hepp, U., Kraemer, B., et al. 2006. "Evidence for Low-grade Systemic Proinflammatory Activity in Patients with Posttraumatic Stress Disorder." *Journal of Psychiatric Research* 41, no. 9: 744-752. http://dx.doi.org/10.1016/j.jpsychires.2006.06.009.

Yeragani, V. K., et al. 1998. "Decreased Heart-period Variability in Patients with Panic Disorder: A Study of Holter ECG Records." *Psychiatry Research* 78: 89-99.

OTHER RESOURCES

The Association for Comprehensive Energy Psychology (ACEP) website provides information for professionals and the public on current energy psychology techniques, research, educational programs, and a referral database of professionals. ACEP has an extensive audio library of past conferences and information on current research in the field of energy psychology. ACEP offers certification programs and an annual international conference in the spring. http://www.energypsych.org.

The Canadian Association for Integrative and Energy Therapies (CAIET) is a nonprofit organization of professionals practicing energy therapies. CAIET provides current information about energy therapies, a referral base for consumers, an annual conference, and opportunities for training and education in energy therapies. https://CAIET.org.

The Chopra Center at La Costa Resort and Spa. In addition to the healing and retreat center, Deepak Chopra, MD, offers online courses, workshops, and practices. He often collaborates with Oprah Winfrey to offer free online meditation programs. https://www.chopra.com/.

Dr. Dan Siegel. Resources on healthy parenting and interpersonal awareness for healthy relationships. http://www.drdansiegel.com/resources.

Dynamic Energetic Healing. An approach integrating various energy psychology modalities. http://www.dynamicenergetichealing.com.

Esalen. A retreat center in Big Sur, California, for healing, learning, and self discovery. https://www.esalen.org.

Vincent Felitti's recorded, full presentation in 2006: https://www.youtube.com/watch?v=Me07G3Erbw8 (shorter presentations are also available).

1440 Multiversity. A retreat center in Scotts Valley, California, whose vision is to foster healing, wellness, and community. https://1440.org.

Friendship Circle. http://www.friendshipcircle.org/blog/2013/01/08/10-causes-of-post-traumatic-stress-disorder-in-children/.

The Guild of Energists. A nonprofit international organization based in the United Kingdom, which offers educational programs and information on professionals practicing energy therapies. https://goe.ac.

Hay House, Inc. A publishing company with self-help books and publications. http://www.hayhouse.com.

Kripalu. A retreat, educational center in the Berkshires, Massachusetts. https://kripalu.org.

National Institute for the Clinical Application of Behavioral Medicine (NICABM). A resource for continuing education for health practitioners; a pioneer in mind-body-spirit healing. Their international programs are user friendly to the lay person. http://www.NICABM.com.

Omega Institute. A retreat center in Rhinebeck, New York, hosting stress reduction and wellness programs and trainings. http://www.eomega.org.

Preventive Medicine Research Institute in Sausalito, California. http://pmri.org and https://www.retreatfinder.com. A website with information on some retreats around the world.

Sensorimotor Psychotherapy. https://www.sensorimotorpsychotherapy.org/index.html.

Sounds True. A publishing house of educational and spiritual books and recordings, in Boulder, CO. http://www.soundstrue.com.

The Stress Reduction Clinic. A mindfulness and stress-reduction program in Shrewsbury, Massachusetts.

MOVIES

Escape Fire: The Fight to Rescue American Healthcare. Aisle C Productions and Our Time Projects, 2012.

Heal. Elevative Entertainment and i2i Productions. http://www.healdocumentary.com.

The Secret. Prime Time Productions and Nine Network Australia, 2007.

Dalai Lama Awakening. Wakan Films, 2014.

What the Bleep Do We Know. Captured Light and Lord of the Wind, 2004.

CDs

Nawang Kerchog. *Tibetan Meditation Music for Quiet Mind and Peaceful Heart.* Sounds True, Boulder, Colorado.

Swami Shankardev Saravasti and Jayne Stevenson: *Introduction to Pranic Healing: Experience of Breath and Energy.* http://www. bigshakti.com.

Devorah Zaslow. *Return Again: Stories of Healing and Renewal.* http://rabbidavidzaslow.com/return-again/.

About the Author

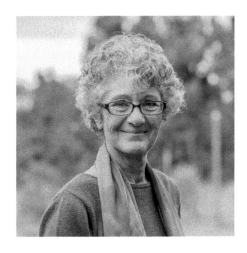

Working as an emergency physician in the greater Boston area, Dr. Joalie Davie has treated thousands of patients and also served on the clinical faculties of Harvard Medical School and the Tufts University School of Medicine. Her expertise is built upon a foundation in standard medical training, having received a BA with honors from Harvard College and an MD from the University of Massachusetts Medical School.

For twenty years, she has integrated holistic therapies in her caregiving, and she continues to dedicate her practice to supporting individuals who seek healing through natural and alternative approaches.

Joalie is the founder and director of Health from Within—a center for healing, wellness, stress reduction, and community. In addition to her private practice, she leads workshops and retreats, situated in pristine locations, for individuals and small groups. To find out more about her work or to contact her, please visit www. HealthFromWithin.org.

Dear Reader

I hope this book has provided validation, encouragement, and support for your journey to health and well-being, that it empowered you and gave you more confidence in your quest for wellness. I have enjoyed sharing these stories of other individuals' journeys along a holistic path—please share them with those in your life who may be exploring their own possibilities for health.

I believe that prevention is key to averting most diseases, whether mental, physical, emotional, or psychological. The answers lie in creating a society that cares, that provides community, and that protects and supports children by helping young families with social programs, safety nets, and educational programs to build social and parenting skills. Only then will there be true prevention and healing.

My wish for you, the reader—and for all people—is the achievement of well-being, good health, and living in a compassionate and loving community.

CPSIA information can be obtained
at www.ICGtesting.com
Printed in the USA
FFHW022332021118
49185763-53399FF